Kerry L. Hull, PhD
Professor, Department of Biology
Bishop's University
Adjunct Professor, Department of Physiology, Faculty of Medicine
University of Sherbrooke
Sherbrooke, Quebec
Canada

Jennifer Shaw, MNS
Assistant Professor
Polk University
Celebration, Florida

ENHANCED FIRST EDITION

Laboratory Manual to Accompany

Human Form | Human Function

Essentials of Anatomy & Physiology

Thomas H. McConnell • Kerry L. Hull

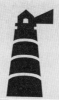

JONES & BARTLETT
LEARNING

World Headquarters
Jones & Bartlett Learning
5 Wall Street
Burlington, MA 01803
978-443-5000
info@jblearning.com
www.jblearning.com

Jones & Bartlett Learning books and products are available through most bookstores and online booksellers. To contact Jones & Bartlett Learning directly, call 800-832-0034, fax 978-443-8000, or visit our website, www.jblearning.com.

Substantial discounts on bulk quantities of Jones & Bartlett Learning publications are available to corporations, professional associations, and other qualified organizations. For details and specific discount information, contact the special sales department at Jones & Bartlett Learning via the above contact information or send an email to specialsales@jblearning.com.

21828-2

Production Credits
VP, Product Management: Amanda Martin
Director of Product Management: Cathy L. Esperti
Product Assistant: Ashley Malone
Product Coordinator: Elena Sorrentino
Digital Project Specialist: Angela Dooley
Director of Marketing: Andrea DeFronzo
Marketing Manager: Suzy Balk
Production Services Manager: Colleen Lamy
VP, Manufacturing and Inventory Control: Therese Connell
Product Fulfillment Manager: Wendy Kilborn
Composition: S4Carlisle Publishing Services
Project Management: S4Carlisle Publishing Services
Cover & Text Design: Michael O'Donnell
Senior Media Development Editor: Troy Liston
Rights Specialist: Becky Damon
Printing and Binding: McNaughton & Gunn

Library of Congress Cataloging-in-Publication Data
Library of Congress Cataloging-in-Publication Data unavailable at time of printing.

LCCN: 2020933350

6048

Printed in the United States of America
24 23 22 21 20   10 9 8 7 6 5 4 3 2 1

Preface

Welcome to the *Laboratory Manual to Accompany Human Form, Human Function Enhanced Edition!*

The *Human Form, Human Function* textbook showcases the human body as a fully integrated organism in which form and function are inseparable, with its own highly developed communication systems. This Laboratory Manual is designed to communicate the *Human Form, Human Function* message by taking students on a journey of hands-on exploration and discovery while reinforcing concepts in both anatomy *and* physiology. The accessible, conversational narrative style of the textbook is also carried through here in the Laboratory Manual.

Laboratory Manual to Accompany Human Form, Human Function is organized to:

- **Connect the laboratories with the textbook.** Following this Preface, you'll find a table that shows at a glance the correlation of labs with the textbook chapters, and on the opening page of each lab, you'll find the textbook correlation as well. When applicable, lab activities use art adapted from the *Human Form, Human Function* figures. Other labs refer students to case studies and figures in the textbook.
- **Prepare students for laboratory.** Each lab begins with a Details table that lists the activities in the lab, the objectives of each activity, the required materials, and estimated time to spend on each activity. Brief Overviews orient students to the overall goals of the activities in the lab. Need to Know lists remind students of concepts and material they should already have mastered before starting on the labs—much like those in the *Human Form, Human Function* textbook. Finally, Pre-Lab Activities "warm up" students for the lab activities that follow.
- **Walk students through laboratory.** This manual contains a variety of activities—some in groups, some with partners, some individual, some very-hands-on, some less so. Yet, each activity is presented consistently with clear instructions and questions, with adequate space to write, color, or draw when necessary.
- **Successfully wrap up each laboratory.** Every lab ends with a Post-Lab Assessment, giving students a few minutes at the end of each lab to cement in their minds the concepts with which they worked that day.

Special Note for Instructors

Lab instructors know that time management is a key issue within each lab period and throughout the semester. *Laboratory Manual to Accompany Human Form, Human Function* includes 27 laboratories containing a total of 135 activities, but we don't expect you to use every single one! We've included so many labs and activities so that you can feel free to pick and choose among them to customize your laboratory based on your students' needs and the time and equipment you have available.

Important resources for instructors include:

- Instructor's Laboratory Guide: available online to all instructors who adopt this text, see this guide for tips on lab set-up as well as information on where to obtain laboratory materials and equipment.
- Answers to the Activity Questions: available online to all instructors so you can check your students' work.
- Dissection Atlas: the online atlas that comes with the *Human Form, Human Function* textbook is available on the Laboratory Manual's website as well.

Please visit the text's online site, or contact your Jones & Barlett Learning Account Representative for for access to the additional online materials.

Correlation of Labs with Textbook Chapters

Contents

1

Anatomical Terminology

Textbook Correlation: Chapter 1—Form, Function, and Life

Details

Activities	Activity Objectives	Required Materials	Estimated Time
1-1: Anatomical Directions	Use anatomical terms in explaining organ/structure relationships.	● Articulated skeleton (optional)	15–20 min
1-2: Body Planes	Identify the body plane that various models/slides are displaying.	● Banana or cucumber (1 per group of 4 students) ● Various models demonstrating body planes (optional; see "Instructor Resources" for ideas)	20 min
1-3: Surface Anatomy	Identify various structures and regions of the body using correct terminology.	● 2 large pieces of butcher paper per group of 2 students ● Scissors ● Tape ● Several pieces of scrap paper	45 min
1-4: General and Specific Body Cavities	Identify the general and specific body cavities on models.	● Articulated skeleton ● Torso model	20 min
1-5: Serous Membranes	Explain the relationship between the serous membrane layers and identify the locations of the membranes	● Balloon	10 min

Overview

Directional terms are used to explain the location of body structures and regions in relation to one another. This is common practice for anatomists and health care providers and is even used in medical dramas, such as *House* or *Grey's Anatomy*. Watch an episode or two and you will hear many of the phrases learned today! For example, instead of stating, "The tumor is above the large intestine," you'll hear the TV physician state, "The tumor is superior to the large intestine." This clarifies that the tumor is close to the large intestine, at the side nearest the head. As another example, a clinician might say that a wound affecting the small intestine is anterior to the kidneys. This is because the small intestine is closer than the kidneys to the front of the body (the kidneys adhere to the dorsal wall, or back, of the body). Think of the difference between a superficial wound and a deep wound. How do the two wounds differ? How would that relate to the body and the relationship between organs? Today's lab will introduce the language of anatomy.

Need to Know

- All anatomical terms reflect a person in the standard anatomical position:
  - Standing up straight
  - Feet flat
  - Palms facing forward

- Directional terms compare the location of two structures:
  - Anterior/Posterior
    - ○ **Anterior:** closer to the front of the body
    - ○ **Posterior:** closer to the back of the body
    - ○ Hint: "A" is closer to the front of the alphabet and "P" is closer to the back of the alphabet
    - ○ Used only for two-legged animals
  - Ventral/Dorsal
    - ○ **Ventral:** closer to the belly of the animal (same as *anterior* in humans)
    - ○ **Dorsal:** closer to the back of the animal (same as *posterior* in humans)
    - ○ Can be used to describe locations in four-legged animals
    - ○ Hint: think about the location of the *dorsal* fin of a dolphin
  - Superior/Inferior
    - ○ **Superior:** closer to the head
    - ○ **Inferior:** closer to the feet
    - ○ Used only for two-legged animals
  - Caudal/Cranial
    - ○ **Cranial:** closer to the head
    - ○ **Caudal:** closer to the tail
    - ○ These terms are more commonly used for four-legged animals
  - Medial/Lateral
    - ○ Imagine a line drawn down the center of your body separating you into two equal right and left halves
    - ○ **Medial:** closer to the midline
    - ○ **Lateral:** further from the midline
  - Proximal/Distal
    - ○ **Proximal:** closer to the point of origin, or attachment
    - ○ **Distal:** further from the point of origin is distal (think distance)
    - ○ Used to describe bones of the appendages (limbs)

- Superficial/Deep
  - ○ **Superficial:** closer to the body surface
  - ○ **Deep:** farther away from the body surface
  - ○ Example: the brain is deep to the skull

- Anatomical planes divide the body into separate regions along imaginary lines.
  - A **transverse plane** separates the superior body from the inferior body.
  - A **sagittal plane** separates the left body from the right body.
  - A **frontal plane** separates the anterior body from the posterior body.
  - An **oblique plane** separates at a diagonal, or angle.

- Regional terms describe different body regions.
  - Example: the lower limb
    - ○ Layperson terms: upper leg, kneecap, shin, ankle, foot, and toes
    - ○ Anatomical terms: femoral region, patellar region, crural region, tarsal region, pedal region, and digital region
  - Practice using these terms at home so that you will remember them!

- The body contains **cavities,** or potential spaces filled with organs.
  - The **dorsal** and **ventral** body cavities are each further divided into specific body cavities.
    - ○ The **cranial** and **spinal** cavities make up the dorsal body cavity.
    - ○ The ventral body cavity is further divided into the **thoracic** and **abdominopelvic** cavities.
    - ○ The abdominopelvic cavity is further divided into the **abdominal** and **pelvic** body cavities.

- **Serous membranes** surround the visceral organs.
  - Composed of two layers:
    - ○ Superficial **parietal** layer, often attached to the body wall.
    - ○ Deeper **visceral** layer, attached to the organ.
    - ○ A space is found between the two layers and is typically filled with fluid.
  - The **pericardium** encompasses the heart.
  - The **pleurae** surround the lungs.
  - The **peritoneum** surrounds most of the organs in the abdominal cavity.

Pre-Lab Activity

Students should complete this activity before completing the lab activities that follow.

1. Label the plane that each image below represents.

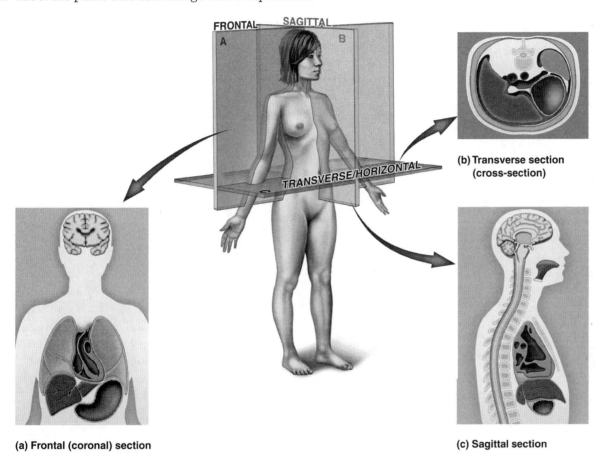

(a) Frontal (coronal) section

(b) Transverse section (cross-section)

(c) Sagittal section

2. Draw arrows on the following images in the direction listed. When drawing the arrow, use the color written next to the direction.
   a. Lateral: purple
   b. Superior: orange
   c. Distal: blue
   d. Anterior: red

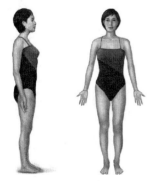

3. Name the serous membrane that surrounds each of the following organs.

    a. Heart: _____

    b. Lungs: _____

    c. Intestines: _____

4. Label each cavity on the figure below and color each cavity according to the color key below:
    a. Abdominal cavity: green
    b. Cranial cavity: purple
    c. Pelvic cavity: red
    d. Spinal cavity: yellow
    e. Thoracic cavity: orange

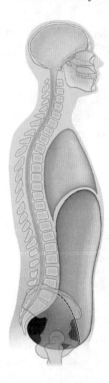

5. Which of the above cavities are considered ventral cavities?

_____

Anatomical Directions

Activity Instructions and Questions

Working in pairs or groups of four, practice using the various anatomical terms by performing the action described in the following questions to come up with the answers.

1. Do the palms face *anteriorly* or *posteriorly* in standard anatomical position? What other term can describe the position of the palms in relation to the backs of the hands?

   _____

2. Obtain an articulated skeleton. If an articulated skeleton is not available, use your own forearm. Grasp the forearm and rotate it so that the palm is facing anteriorly and then so that the palm is facing posteriorly. Watch the bones of the forearm. Record your observations.

   _____

   _____

   _____

3. When explaining which forearm bone is medial, does it matter which way the palm should face? Explain using anatomical terms.

   _____

   _____

   _____

4. Practice using the anatomical terms in the "Need to Know" with your partner, pointing out examples on yourself and/or your partner. Write your examples in the spaces below.

   _____

   _____

   _____

   _____

Activity 1-2

Body Planes

Body planes are important in different types of imaging tests, such as a CT, MRI, or ultrasound scan. The technician must understand the view, or plane, ordered by the physician in order to properly position the body and obtain appropriate images of the desired organ. It's also essential to understand planes if you are to study models and slides, or when you're dissecting. We will use a banana or cucumber to simulate the various body planes prior to visualizing them on models. You can also see the body planes in Figure 1.11 in your textbook.

Activity Instructions and Questions

Work in a group of four students and obtain either a banana or cucumber for each member of the group. Then perform the tasks described below to come up with your answers.

1. Cut one object (banana or cucumber) in half horizontally, separating the top from the bottom. What plane is demonstrated when you make this cut? Explain your answer.

   _____

   _____

2. Cut the second object in half vertically, separating the right side from the left side. Identify the plane demonstrated when you make this cut.

   _____

3. Cut the third object in half vertically, separating the front of the object from the back of the object. What plane are you observing? Explain your answer.

   _____

   _____

4. Cut the fourth object in a diagonal direction (halfway through the fruit or veggie). Identify the plane that you are observing.

   _____

Optional Activity

If models are available, practice by determining the plane that is demonstrated by the model. Fill in the following table.

Table 1.1 Planes Demonstrated on Models	
Model	**Plane Demonstrated by Model**

Activity 1-3

Surface Anatomy

Activity Instructions

Work in groups of two.

1. Cut several pieces of scrap paper into many small squares.

2. Write each of the following surface anatomical terms on a small square of paper (one term per square).

Anterior Surface Terms

- Antebrachial
- Antecubital
- Axillary
- Brachial
- Buccal
- Carpal
- Cervical
- Coxal
- Crural
- Digital
- Femoral
- Inguinal
- Mammary
- Mental
- Nasal
- Oral
- Orbital
- Otic
- Palmar
- Patellar
- Pedal
- Pubic
- Sternal
- Tarsal
- Umbilical

Posterior Surface Terms

- Acromial
- Calcaneal
- Cephalic
- Femoral
- Gluteal
- Lumbar
- Manual
- Occipital
- Olecranal
- Plantar
- Popliteal
- Sacral
- Scapular
- Sural
- Vertebral

3. Obtain two large pieces of butcher paper.

4. Draw or trace a picture of the anterior surface of the human body. One student may wish to trace the outline of the second student.

5. Repeat step 4, but this time draw the posterior surface of the human body.

6. Work with your partner and tape each of the surface terms on the drawings/tracings of the body, both on the anterior side and the posterior side. Do not refer to your textbook, just try to do the best you can from memory.

7. After placing each term on the drawn/traced body, refer to Figure 1.12 in your textbook to check your answers. Move any wrong terms to the correct area of the body.

Activity Questions

Fill in the blanks using surface anatomy terms:

1. The correct term for the armpit is the _____ area.

2. The correct term for the neck is the _____ area.

3. The correct term for the back of the knee is the _____ area.

4. The area on the arm in which blood is typically drawn is the _____ area.

5. The bottom of the foot is known as the _____ area.

General and Specific Body Cavities

Activity Instructions and Questions

The goal of this activity is to identify the general and specific body cavities on an articulated skeleton and a torso model. As you answer the questions below, use general terms in describing the bones.

1. Obtain an articulated skeleton and a torso model. Take all of the organs out of the torso model and place them in a pile.

2. Identify the cranial cavity and the spinal cavity on the skeleton. What is the large group of bones that forms the cranial cavity? Which collection of bones forms the spinal cavity?

   _____

   _____

3. Use the torso model to identify the thoracic cavity and the abdominopelvic cavity. These cavities can also be observed in the articulated skeleton. Which bones form the thoracic cavity?

   _____

4. The abdominopelvic cavity can be further separated into the abdominal cavity and the pelvic cavity. Locate both cavities on both the torso model and the articulated skeleton. Which bones form the pelvic cavity?

   _____

5. **Critical Thinking:** The abdominal cavity is not protected by bone. Discuss the ramifications if it were to have a bony enclosure. Then identify a drawback of an abdominal cavity without a bony enclosure.

   _____

   _____

   _____

6. Name the organ (muscle) that separates the thoracic cavity from the abdominopelvic cavity.

   _____

7. When you have completed this activity, don't forget to put the organs back in the torso model.

Activity 1-5

Serous Membranes

A partially inflated balloon will be used to demonstrate the serous membranes. See Figure 1.14 and in your textbook for more information about how these membranes form.

Activity Instructions

1. Obtain a balloon and blow it up slightly. Tie it off.

2. Place your fist in the partially blown-up balloon (do not pop the balloon).

3. Observe how the balloon surrounds your fist. Your fist represents an organ, and two layers of the balloon represent the serous membranes.

Activity Questions

1. If your fist is the heart and the balloon is the serous membrane surrounding the heart, name the membrane touching your fist. Be specific, and explain your answer.

_____

_____

_____

2. If your fist were the lung, name the most superficial membrane. Be specific, and explain your answer.

_____

_____

_____

3. **Critical Thinking:** The serous membranes surround hard-working organs that constantly move in relation to other organs. Explain your understanding of the purposes of the serous membranes.

_____

_____

_____

Post-Lab Assessment

1. Which plane separates the ventral portion of the body from the dorsal portion of the body?

_____

2. Which plane separates the superior portion of the body from the inferior portion of the body?

_____

3. The urinary bladder is _____ to the rectum.

4. The stomach is _____ to the small intestine.

5. The back of the knee is called the _____ area.

6. The palms of the hands face _____ when the body is in standard anatomical position.

7. Name the two specific cavities found within the dorsal cavity.

_____

8. The heart is _____ to the lungs.

9. The carpals (wrist bones) are _____ to the humerus (upper arm bone).

10. Bone is _____ to skeletal muscle.

11. The brain is _____ to the spinal cord.

12. The kidneys are _____ to the small intestine.

13. The rib cage is _____ to the lungs.

2

Organ System Overview

Textbook Correlation: Chapter 1—Form, Function, and Life

Details

Activities	Activity Objectives	Required Materials	Estimated Time
2-1: Organ Identification	Identify the major organs of the body.	● Torso model ● Pelvic models ● Brain model	45–60 min
2-2: Body Cavities and Organs	Determine the cavities (both general and specific) in which each organ is found.	● Models used in 2-1 ● Stickers of various colors (green, red, brown, yellow, black, purple, blue, pink, orange, gray, white, and peach)	20–30 min
2-3: Organ System Practice	Apply the knowledge gained in previous lab activities	● None	5 min

Overview

Justin, a healthy 17-year-old male, was rushed to the hospital after complaining of severe abdominal pain during football practice. He also mentioned pain in his left shoulder. Upon admission, his blood pressure was 95/62 and his heart rate was 87 beats per minute. The EMT reported that Justin had received a severe blow to the abdominal area during practice. The ER doctors rushed Justin to the OR and an immediate splenectomy (removal of the spleen) was performed. Several days later, as Justin was recovering from surgery, he had several questions such as these: *Where, exactly, is the spleen? What does it look like? What does it do? Will I be okay without one?*

Upon completion of the lab activities, you will be able to answer the questions about the spleen as well as many other major body organs. This lab will also make watching medical TV shows much more enjoyable, since you will understand the structure and location of the organs discussed.

Need to Know

- Organisms, such as humans, are made up of organ systems, which are in turn made up of organs.

- Organs are composed of two or more types of tissue.

- Tissues are collections of cells with similar structure and therefore similar function.

- Cells are made up of molecules, which are groups of atoms bonded together.

- Today's lab activity will focus on the 11 organ systems found in the human body and the organs they contain:
  - Cardiovascular system
  - Digestive system
  - Endocrine system
  - Integumentary system
  - Lymphatic system
  - Male reproductive system/female reproductive system
  - Muscular system
  - Nervous system
  - Respiratory system
  - Skeletal system
  - Urinary system

Pre-Lab Activity

Students should complete this activity before completing the lab activities that follow. You can use Figure 1.6 in your textbook for reference.

Match the correct organ system with its function, by writing the correct letters in the blanks.

_____ 1. Responsible for electrical communication throughout the body.

_____ 2. Regulates blood volume and rids the body of nitrogenous wastes.

_____ 3. Contains the largest organ of the body as well as hair, and nails.

_____ 4. Produces and secretes chemicals, called hormones, involved in communication.

_____ 5. Contains hard organs that protect delicate organs such as the brain, spinal cord, heart, and lungs.

_____ 6. Contains a copulatory organ and another organ that produces sperm and secretes testosterone.

_____ 7. Contains a pump and a blood transport system; each contraction of the pump moves the blood through the transport system in order to drop off nutrients and pick up wastes.

_____ 8. Transfers fluid from the extracellular spaces to the bloodstream.

_____ 9. Draws air into the body and releases air into the environment.

_____ 10. Moves bones.

_____ 11. Breaks down ingested nutrients for energy production or for storage.

_____ 12. Contains a copulatory organ and another organ that produces oocytes (eggs), estrogens, and progesterone.

A. Cardiovascular system
B. Digestive system
C. Endocrine system
D. Female reproductive system
E. Integumentary system
F. Lymphatic system
G. Male reproductive system
H. Muscular system
I. Nervous system
J. Respiratory system
K. Skeletal system
L. Urinary system

Organ Identification

Activity Instructions

Use Figure 1.6 in the text to help you with this activity.

1. Take the organs out of the torso model and identify each organ (listed below) as you remove it. Some of the organs cannot be removed, but you are still responsible for identifying them in the torso model.

- Adrenal glands
- Anus
- Bone
- Brain
- Bronchi
- Diaphragm
- Ductus deferens
- Esophagus
- Gallbladder
- Kidneys
- Large intestine
- Larynx
- Liver
- Lungs
- Muscle
- Nasal cavity
- Oral cavity
- Ovaries
- Pancreas
- Penis
- Pharynx
- Pineal gland
- Pituitary gland
- Prostate
- Rectum
- Skin
- Small intestine
- Spinal cord
- Spleen
- Stomach
- Testes
- Thyroid
- Trachea
- Ureters
- Urethra
- Urinary bladder
- Uterine tubes
- Uterus
- Vagina

2. Use the color code below and place the correct color sticker on each organ to correspond with the correct organ system. (Note: some organs are part of more than one organ system, so put all colors that apply on those organs.)

- Respiratory system: green
- Cardiovascular system: red
- Integumentary system: purple
- Digestive system: brown
- Urinary system: yellow
- Endocrine system: black
- Male reproductive system: blue
- Female reproductive system: pink
- Lymphatic system: orange
- Skeletal system: peach
- Muscular system: white
- Nervous system: gray

Activity Questions

Put the correct letter of the organ system or systems next to the corresponding organ using your labeled organs above.

_____ Adrenal glands

_____ Anus

_____ Bone

_____ Brain

_____ Bronchi

_____ Diaphragm

_____ Ductus deferens

_____ Esophagus

_____ Gallbladder

_____ Kidneys

_____ Large intestine

_____ Larynx

_____ Liver

_____ Lungs

_____ Muscle

_____ Nasal cavity

_____ Oral cavity

_____ Ovaries

_____ Pancreas

_____ Penis

_____ Pharynx

_____ Pineal gland

_____ Pituitary gland

_____ Prostate

_____ Rectum

_____ Skin

_____ Small intestine

_____ Spinal cord

_____ Spleen

_____ Stomach

_____ Testes

_____ Thyroid

_____ Trachea

_____ Ureters

_____ Urethra

_____ Urinary bladder

_____ Uterine tubes

_____ Uterus

_____ Vagina

A. Cardiovascular system
B. Digestive system
C. Endocrine system
D. Female reproductive system
E. Integumentary system
F. Lymphatic system
G. Male reproductive system
H. Muscular system
I. Nervous system
J. Respiratory system
K. Skeletal system
L. Urinary system

Body Cavities and Organs

Activity Instructions and Questions

Review the information about body cavities in Lab 1. The general body cavities are the dorsal and ventral body cavities. The cranial, spinal, thoracic, abdominal, and pelvic cavities are specific body cavities. Use Figure 1.15 in your textbook to help you with this activity.

1. Look at the organs that cannot be removed from the torso model. Determine the general and specific cavity for each organ and write the appropriate letters for each organ listed below.

2. As you put the other organs back in the torso model, match the correct general and specific cavity for each organ listed below. Write the letter corresponding to the general cavity on the first blank line and the specific cavity on the second blank line for each organ.

_____ _____ Adrenal glands   _____ _____ Pituitary gland

_____ _____ Anus   _____ _____ Prostate

_____ _____ Brain   _____ _____ Rectum

_____ _____ Bronchi   _____ _____ Small intestine

_____ _____ Esophagus   _____ _____ Spinal cord

_____ _____ Gallbladder   _____ _____ Spleen

_____ _____ Kidneys   _____ _____ Stomach

_____ _____ Large intestine   _____ _____ Ureters

_____ _____ Liver   _____ _____ Urethra

_____ _____ Lungs   _____ _____ Urinary bladder

_____ _____ Ovaries   _____ _____ Uterine tubes

_____ _____ Pancreas   _____ _____ Uterus

_____ _____ Pineal gland   _____ _____ Vagina

A. Dorsal body cavity
B. Ventral body cavity
C. Cranial cavity
D. Spinal cavity
E. Thoracic cavity
F. Abdominal cavity
G. Pelvic cavity

Organ System Practice

Activity Instructions and Questions

Applying your knowledge of organ locations and body cavities, circle the correct response.

1. Which one of the following organs is part of the lymphatic system?
   a. Pancreas
   b. Spleen
   c. Adrenal glands
   d. Urinary bladder

2. Which one of the following organs is found in the dorsal body cavity?
   a. Pineal gland
   b. Adrenal gland
   c. Stomach
   d. Urinary bladder

3. Which one of the following organs separates the thoracic cavity from the abdominal cavity?
   a. Liver
   b. Lungs
   c. Diaphragm
   d. Stomach

4. Choose the best pairing regarding the lungs:
   a. Dorsal, thoracic
   b. Ventral, thoracic
   c. Ventral, abdominal
   d. Dorsal, cranial

5. Which of the following organs is found in the pelvic cavity?
   a. Urinary bladder
   b. Kidneys
   c. Spleen
   d. Pancreas

Post-Lab Assessment

1. Name the specific cavity that houses the spleen.

   _____

2. Name the organ system that includes bone.

   _____

3. Name one organ that is part of the nervous system.

   _____

4. Name the organ system that includes the ductus deferens.

   _____

5. Name the general cavity that includes the spinal cord.

   _____

3

Selected Concepts in Chemistry

Textbook Correlation: Chapter 2—Chemistry in Context

Details

Activities	Activity Objectives	Required Materials (per group of 4 students)	Estimated Time
3-1: Measuring pH	• Determine the pH of several substances. • Determine the relative strengths of acids and bases.	• 8 test tubes • Test tube rack • Wax pencil • Eight 20-mL graduated cylinders • 8 pH indicator strips • Test tube brushes	10 min
3-2: Testing for Presence of Organic Compounds	• Identify the organic compounds present in various known substances by using reagents. • Explain the function of a reagent. • Differentiate between quantative and qualitative tests. • Identify the organic compounds present in various unknown substances by using reagents. • Identify the unknown substances through scientific exploration and observation.	• Avocado slice • Special K Vitamin Water • Saltine cracker • Egg albumin • Apple juice • Whole milk • 6 test tubes • Test tube rack • Wax pencil • 4 graduated cylinders • One 250-mL beaker • Hot plate • Test tube clamp • Test tube brush • Well (spot) plate • Wax paper or brown paper bag • Several unknowns • Benedict's reagent • Biuret reagent • Iodine	45 min

Details *(Continued)*

Activities	Activity Objectives	Required Materials (per group of 4 students)	Estimated Time
3-3: Amylase Action on Various Organic Compounds	● Explain enzyme specificity.	● 12 test tubes ● 410-mL graduated cylinders ● One 250-mL beaker ● Wax pencil ● Hot plate ● Boiling beads ● Test tube tongs ● Test tube brush ● Iodine ● Benedict's reagent ● Starch solution ● Albumin solution ● Glucose solution ● 100% amylase	20–30 min
3-4: Effect of Enzyme Concentration on Amylase Effectiveness	● Explain the effect of enzyme concentration on enzyme effectiveness. ● Explain how time affects enzyme action.	● 4 test tubes ● Five 10-mL graduated cylinders ● One 250-mL beaker ● Wax pencil ● Hot plate ● Boiling beads ● Test tube brush ● Benedict's reagent ● Starch solution ● Amylase solutions: [100%], [50%], [10%], [0%]	20–30 min

Overview

Have you ever taken a bite of something sour, such as a lemon, and wondered why it tasted like that? Or have you ever wondered what is in some of your favorite foods? Have you ever thought about how certain foods are broken down in your digestive system? Today's lab activities will answer some of these questions.

Need to Know

● The pH scale expresses how acidic or alkaline (basic) a solution is; that is, it reflects the hydrogen ion (H^+) concentration of the solution. The scale runs from 0 to 14.
  ● **Acids** increase the concentration of H^+ ions in a solution.
    ○ Stronger acids liberate more H^+ and have a lower pH (lower than 7).
    ○ Example: orange juice (pH 3.6) is acidic.

- **Bases**, or alkaline substances, reduce the concentration of H^+ in a solution.
  - Many bases release OH^- ions, which react with H^+ to form H_2O (water).
  - Stronger bases absorb more H^+ and have a higher pH (higher than 7).
  - Example: apple juice (pH 8.0) is alkaline.
- **Neutral substances: pH is 7.0**
  - The concentration of H^+ is equal to the concentration of OH^-.
  - Example: pure (distilled) water is neutral.
- The pH scale is *logarithmic*: an increase (or decrease) of 1 pH unit equals a 10-fold difference in strength.
  - Example: a solution with a pH of 2.0 is 10 times more acidic than a solution with a pH of 3.0.
  - Example: a substance with a pH of 2.0 is 100 times (10×10) more acidic than a substance with a pH of 4.0.

- Foods contain one or more **nutrients.**
  - **Proteins**
    - Composed of amino acids bound together by peptide bonds.
    - Dietary examples: meats and beans.
    - Cells use amino acids to build needed structural and functional proteins.
  - **Lipids**
    - A broad group of compounds that are insoluble in water.
    - Triglycerides ("fats") are common dietary lipids and the primary lipid storage form in the body.
    - Cholesterol is a type of lipid called a *steroid*.
    - Lipid-rich foods include egg yolks, nuts, meat, dairy products, and plant oils.
    - Lipids are used for energy, insulation, chemical signals, and to construct cell membranes.
  - **Carbohydrates**
    - Monosaccharides (e.g., glucose) contain one sugar molecule.
    - Disaccharides (e.g., lactose) contain two sugar molecules.
    - Polysaccharides (e.g., starch, glycogen) contain many sugar molecules. Monosaccharides are used to generate ATP; polysaccharides are used to store carbohydrates.

- **Enzymes** are proteins that play critical roles in cell function.
  - **Catabolic** enzymes (such as digestive enzymes) break down complex molecules into simpler molecules.
    - Example: glycogen (polysaccharide) → glucose (monosaccharide)
  - **Anabolic** enzymes assemble simple molecules into more complex ones.
    - Example: amino acids → protein

- **Reagents:** indicate the presence of various organic compounds by changing color.
  - **Negative result:** the organic compound tested for is not present.
  - **Positive result:** the organic compound tested for is present.
  - **Qualitative reagents** indicate whether or not an organic compound is present.
  - **Quantitative reagents** indicate how much of the organic compound is present.
  - Three reagents will be used today. Please refer to Table 3.1 for interpretation of reagent data.
    - Benedict's reagent tests for the presence of glucose.
    - Iodine tests for the presence of starch.
    - Biuret reagent tests for the presence of protein.

Table 3.1 Reagent Information

Reagent	Organic Compound Detected	Negative Result	Positive Result	Type of Test
Benedict's reagent	Glucose	Blue	Green (low glucose concentration) → yellow → orange → red (high glucose concentration)	Quantitative
Iodine	Starch	Brown	Purple or Black	Qualitative
Biuret reagent	Protein	Blue	Purple	Qualitative

Pre-Lab Activity

Students should complete this activity before completing the lab activities that follow.

Activity Instructions

Match the following terms with the correct statement below. Some answers may used more than once.

_____ 1. A type of monosaccharide that is used to make ATP

_____ 2. Dissociates H^+ ions

_____ 3. A test that can measure the amount of a chemical present

_____ 4. A substance that increases the rate of a chemical reaction without becoming part of the product

_____ 5. Any chemical that detects the presence of specific organic compounds

_____ 6. A test that determines the presence but not the amount of specific compounds

_____ 7. A type of polysaccharide that is found in toast

_____ 8. Dissociates OH^- ions

_____ 9. Example of a pH reading of 6.7

A. Acid
B. Base
C. Enzyme
D. Glucose
E. Qualitative test
F. Quantitative test
G. Reagent
H. Starch

Measuring pH

This activity measures the pH of different substances.

Activity Instructions

1. Obtain 8 test tubes and label them from 1 to 8 using a wax pencil.

2. Place the test tubes in the test tube rack.

3. Use a graduated cylinder to pour approximately 10 to 15 mL of tomato juice into test tube 1.

4. Use a **different** graduated cylinder to pour approximately 10 to 15 mL of simulated blood into test tube 2.

5. Repeat the above instructions* for the other tubes, as follows:
   - Test tube 3: simulated urine
   - Test tube 4: distilled water
   - Test tube 5: ammonia
   - Test tube 6: baking soda
   - Test tube 7: vinegar
   - Test tube 8: glass cleaner

6. Obtain 8 pH indicator strips.

7. Dip one indicator strip into each of the test tubes. Be sure to use a new indicator strip in each test tube in order to prevent cross-contamination.

8. Remove the indicator strips one by one, recording the results of each in Table 3.2 on the following page. Use the key on the pH strip bottle to interpret the color changes.

9. Throw away the indicator strips and pour the test tube contents down the sink.

10. Wash the test tubes with the test tube brushes and return them to the test tube rack.

Be sure to use a different graduated cylinder for measuring each substance in order to prevent cross-contamination.

Table 3.2 pH Measurement Data		
Test Tube Number	**Contents**	**pH**
1	Tomato juice	
2	Simulated blood	
3	Simulated urine	
4	Distilled water	
5	Ammonia	
6	Baking soda	
7	Vinegar	
8	Glass cleaner	

Activity Questions

1. What is the most acidic substance (the strongest acid)?

_____

2. What is the weakest acid?

_____

3. What is the most alkaline substance (the strongest base)?

_____

4. Which substance is neutral? What does that mean?

_____

_____

5. Choose the correct statement regarding the pH of blood:
   a. It is a weak acid.
   b. It is a strong acid.
   c. It is a weak base.
   d. It is a strong base.

6. How much weaker was the baking soda compared with the ammonia? Explain in terms of the quantity of dissociated hydroxyl anions as well as logarithmically.

_____

_____

_____

_____

Activity 3-2

Testing for the Presence of Organic Compounds

This lab activity tests various foods and liquids for the presence of carbohydrates (glucose or starch), lipids, or protein. Various reagents will be used. Please refer back to Table 3.1 (Reagent Information) when interpreting your data. Remember that a positive result means that the organic substance is present and a negative result means that the organic substance is not present.

You will first test a group of "known" substances for organic compound constituents. Then you will test a series of "unknown" substances for the presence of organic compounds. You'll also observe color, shape, and texture in order to determine each substance's identity—just like a food detective.

Activity Instructions: Glucose Test

1. Obtain 6 test tubes, a wax pencil, and a test tube rack. Label the test tubes 1 to 6 with the wax pencil.

2. For samples 1 and 3, place a small piece of each solid into the correct test tube. For the other samples, use a graduated cylinder to pour approximately 10 mL of each liquid into the tube. Use a different graduated cylinder for each liquid so that you do not cross-contaminate.
   1. Avocado (small piece)
   2. Special K Vitamin Water
   3. Saltine cracker (small piece)
   4. Egg albumin (egg white)

5. Apple juice
6. Whole milk

3. Fill a 250-mL beaker approximately half full of tap water.

4. Place the 250-mL beaker on the hot plate and heat to a boil.

5. While waiting for the water to boil, put several drops of Benedict's reagent into all 6 test tubes.

6. Once the water comes to a boil, place the first 3 test tubes in the beaker.

7. Watch and observe for a color change. (Note: a brown color indicates that the test tube was in the water bath for too long and the glucose has burned.)

8. Record the color of each test tube in Table 3.3: Glucose Test Results.

9. Remove the test tubes with the test tube clamps and place them in the test tube rack.

10. Repeat instructions 6 to 8 with test tubes 4 to 6.

11. Wait for the test tubes to cool, then pour the contents down the drain (liquids) or place them in the trash (solids).

12. Clean the test tubes with the test tube brush.

Table 3.3 Glucose Test Results			
Test Tube Number	Contents	Color After Heat Was Added	Was Glucose Present?
1	Avocado		
2	Special K Vitamin Water		
3	Saltine cracker		
4	Egg albumin		
5	Apple juice		
6	Whole milk		

Activity Instructions: Protein Test

1. Obtain 6 test tubes, a wax pencil, and a test tube rack.

2. Label the test tubes 1 to 6 with the wax pencil.

3. For samples 1 and 3, place a small piece of each solid into the correct test tube. For the other samples, use a graduated cylinder to pour approximately 10 mL of each liquid into the tube. Use a different graduated cylinder for each liquid so that you do not cross-contaminate.
   1. Avocado (small piece)
   2. Special K Vitamin Water
   3. Saltine cracker (small piece)

4. Egg albumin (egg white)
5. Apple juice
6. Whole milk

4. Put a few drops (3 or 4) of biuret reagent in each test tube.

5. Observe the test tubes for a color change (blue to purple).

6. Record your observations in Table 3.4: Protein Test Results.

7. Pour the liquids down the drain and place the solids in the trash.

8. Clean the test tubes with the test tube brush.

Table 3.4	Protein Test Results		
Test Tube Number	**Contents**	**Color After Reagent Was Added**	**Was Protein Present?**
1	Avocado		
2	Special K Vitamin Water		
3	Saltine cracker		
4	Egg albumin		
5	Apple juice		
6	Whole milk		

Activity Instructions: Starch Test

1. Obtain a well (spot) plate and a wax pencil.

2. Label the wells 1 to 6 with the wax pencil.

3. Place one substance in each well.
1. Avocado (small piece)
2. Special K Vitamin Water
3. Saltine cracker (small piece)
4. Egg albumin (egg white)
5. Apple juice
6. Whole milk

4. Put a few drops (3 or 4) of iodine in each well. Be careful, because iodine stains skin and clothes.

5. Observe for a color change (brown to dark purple or black) and record the results in Table 3.5: Starch Test Results.

6. Remove the solids from the well plates and place them in the trash.

7. Pour the liquids into the sink and clean the plates.

Table 3.5 Starch Test Results			
Well Number	**Contents**	**Color After Reagent Was Added**	**Was Starch Present?**
1	Avocado		
2	Special K Vitamin Water		
3	Saltine cracker		
4	Egg albumin		
5	Apple juice		
6	Whole milk		

Activity Instructions: Lipid Test

The test for the presence of lipids does not require a reagent. Rather, you'll be observing whether or not the substance leaves a mark on paper. When lipids, or fats, are rubbed on wax paper or a brown paper bag, they leave an opaque or "greasy" mark on the paper. For example, if you place potato chips on a brown paper bag while you're snacking on them, a greasy mark will be left on the paper bag when you finish eating them. That "greasy" or opaque appearance is what you will be looking for in testing the substances for the presence of lipids.

1. Obtain a piece of wax paper or a part of a brown paper bag.

2. Use a pen to divide the paper into six boxes. Number the corners of the boxes from 1 to 6.

3. For samples 1 and 3, rub the solid against the paper in the corresponding box. For the other samples, place a few drops of the liquid in the corresponding box.
   1. Avocado (small piece)
   2. Special K Vitamin Water
   3. Saltine cracker (small piece)
   4. Egg albumin (egg white)
   5. Apple juice
   6. Whole milk

4. Let the paper dry. Observe the paper for the presence of opacity (a greasy spot), which indicates a lipid.

5. Record your observations in Table 3.6: Lipid Test Results.

Table 3.6 Lipid Test Results

Number on Paper	Contents	Appearance: Opaque or Color (once dry)	Were Lipids Present?
1	Avocado		
2	Special K Vitamin Water		
3	Saltine cracker		
4	Egg albumin		
5	Apple juice		
6	Whole milk		

Activity Instructions: Tests for Unknowns

In this part of the activity, you will test several unknown foods and liquids. Each substance should be tested separately for the presence of glucose, protein, starch, and lipids, following the procedures outlined above.

1. Look at each of the unknowns and record color/texture information in Table 3.7: Test Results for Unknowns.

2. Obtain a sample (10 mL of liquids, small part of solid) of each of the unknowns and place each in a separate test tube.

3. Follow the activity instructions for the glucose test and record your results in Table 3.7.

4. Obtain a sample (10 mL of liquid, small part of solid) of each of the unknowns and place each in a separate test tube.

5. Follow the activity instructions for the protein test and record your results in Table 3.7.

6. Obtain a sample (10 mL of liquid, small part of solid) of each of the unknowns and place each in a separate well plate.

7. Follow the activity instructions for the starch test and record your results in Table 3.7.

8. Get a new piece of wax paper or brown paper bag and divide it into boxes according to the number of unknowns.

9. Follow the activity instructions for the lipid test and record your results in Table 3.7.

Table 3.7 Test Results for Unknowns	Unknown 1	Unknown 2	Unknown 3	Unknown 4	Unknown 5
Color					
Texture/consistency					
Color after glucose test					
Color after protein test					
Color after starch test					
Appearance after lipid test					

Activity Questions

1. Which substances tested positive for glucose (contained glucose)?

_____

_____

2. Which substance(s) had the most glucose? How do you know?

_____

_____

3. Of the substances that tested positive for glucose, which has the least amount of glucose? How do you know?

_____

_____

4. Which substances contain protein? How do you know?

_____

_____

5. Which substances contain starch? How do you know?

_____

_____

6. Which substances contain lipids? How do you know?

_____

_____

7. Critical Thinking: After reviewing the data you filled into Table 3.7, state below your hypothesis for the identity of each unknown substance. Explain your reasoning based on data (both observations and test results).

_____

_____

_____

_____

_____

_____

_____

_____

_____

_____

_____

_____

_____

_____

Amylase Action on Various Organic Compounds

Most enzymes have specific active sites that bind to specific substrates (substances) that participate in the reaction catalyzed by enzymes. In today's lab activity, you will test the specificity of an enzyme called amylase, which converts starch into glucose. You will investigate the ability of amylase to change the chemical constituents of three different substances: starch, albumin (egg white), and glucose.

Please refer back to Table 3.1 (Reagent Information) to interpret your results.

Activity Instructions: Control

This part of the activity measures the amount of starch and glucose in the three test substances *before* the addition of amylase.

1. Obtain 3 clean test tubes and number the test tubes 1 to 3, using a wax pencil.

2. Measure (using the graduated cylinder) 10 mL of starch solution and put it in test tube 1.

3. Measure 10 mL of albumin solution and place it in test tube 2. Be sure to use a different graduated cylinder in order to prevent cross-contamination.

4. Measure 10 mL of glucose solution and place it in test tube 3 (use a third graduated cylinder).

5. Test for the presence of starch by adding several drops of iodine to each test tube swirling the tube.

6. Record your observations in Table 3.8 below.

7. Obtain 3 clean test tubes and number the test tubes 4 to 6, using a wax pencil.

8. Measure 10 mL of starch solution and place it in test tube 4.

9. Repeat, using 10 mL of albumin and then 10 mL of glucose and placing the solutions in test tubes 5 and 6, respectively. Be sure to use three different graduated cylinders for each solution in order to prevent cross-contamination.

10. Test for the presence of glucose by adding several drops of Benedict's reagent to each of the three test tubes.

11. Fill a 250-mL beaker halfway with water (tap water is fine) and place on a hot plate. Add boiling beads if available.

12. Bring water to a boil.

13. Place test tubes 4 to 6 in the beaker of boiling water. (Note: Do not leave the test tubes in the boiling water for too long. If the solution turns brown, it has been in the boiling water for too long.)

14. Watch for color changes and record your observations in Table 3.8. A positive result indicates that glucose is present.

Table 3.8 Control		
Organic Compound	**Is Starch Present?**	**Is Glucose Present?**
Starch		
Albumin		
Glucose		

Activity Instructions: Experiment

In this part of the activity, you will see if amylase is capable of changing the chemical constituents of the three test substances.

1. Obtain 3 clean test tubes and number the test tubes 7 to 9, using a wax pencil.

2. Measure 10 mL of starch solution and place it in test tube 7.

3. Repeat, using 10 mL of albumin and 10 mL of glucose, placing in test tubes 8 and 9 (using a different graduated cylinder for each solution).

4. Add 4 mL (using a different graduated cylinder) of 100% amylase to test tubes 7 to 9 and swirl.

5. Let sit for several minutes.

6. Test for the presence of starch, by adding several drops of iodine to each tube. Record your results in Table 3.9 below.

7. Measure 10 mL of starch solution and place it in test tube 10. Repeat, using 10 mL of albumin and 10 mL of glucose in tubes 11 and 12 (respectively).

8. Add 4 mL of 100% amylase to each tube and swirl. Let sit for several minutes.

9. Test for the presence of glucose by following steps 10 to 13 listed above.

10. Watch for color changes and record your observations in Table 3.9 below.

Table 3.9 Organic Compounds + Amylase		
Organic Compound	**Is Starch Present?**	**Is Glucose Present?**
Starch		
Albumin		
Glucose		

Activity Instructions: Cleanup

11. Dump contents of all test tubes in the sink. **Caution: test tubes may be hot!** If the tubes are hot, remove them using test tube tongs.

12. Clean the test tubes with a test tube brush.

13. Place the test tubes in a test tube rack to dry.

Activity Questions

1. Compare your results in Tables 3.8 and 3.9. Did amylase alter the results for the starch sample? Explain.

_____

_____

2. Comparing your results in Tables 3.8 and 3.9, did amylase change the chemical constituents of the glucose sample? Explain your results.

_____

_____

3. Comparing your results in Tables 3.8 and 3.9, did amylase change the chemical constituents of the albumin sample? Explain your results.

_____

_____

_____

4. Based on what you know about organic compounds, explain your results. Be sure to include the mechanism and action of enzymes.

_____

_____

_____

_____

_____

_____

_____

The Effect of Enzyme Concentration on the Effectiveness of Amylase

As seen in Activity 3-3, enzymes have specificity for the reactions they catalyze. Another factor that determines enzyme effectiveness is the concentration of the enzyme present. This lab activity will explore the concept that the concentration of the enzyme affects the rate of the chemical reaction.

Please refer back to Table 3.1 (Reagent Information) in interpreting your results.

Activity Instructions: Control

1. Read steps 2 to 9 below before beginning.

2. Measure 10 mL of starch solution, using a graduated cylinder, and pour it into a test tube.

3. Add 5 mL of 100% amylase to the test tube. Use a different graduated cylinder to pour the amylase in order to prevent cross-contamination.

4. Swirl the test tube and let it sit for 5 minutes.

5. Fill the 250-mL beaker approximately half full with water (tap water is fine).

6. Place the beaker on the hot plate (add boiling beads) and heat to a boil.

7. Put a few drops of Benedict's reagent in the test tube.

8. Place the test tube in the beaker and observe for a color change.

9. Record your observations in Table 3.10 below.

Table 3.10 Organic Compounds + Amylase + Benedict's Reagent		
Organic Compound	**Color After Addition of Iodine**	**Positive (+) or Negative (−) Result**
Starch		
Albumin		
Glucose		

Activity Instructions: Experiment

1. Repeat the procedure above but instead of using 100% amylase, replace with 50% amylase solution, then again with 10% amylase solution and, last, with 0% amylase. These can run concurrently; just be sure to label the test tubes with a wax pencil.

2. Record your observations in Table 3.11 below.

Table 3.11 Amylase Concentration Data	
Amylase Concentration	**Color After Adding Heat**
100% Amylase	
50% Amylase	
10% Amylase	
0% Amylase	

Activity Instructions: Cleanup

1. Dump contents of all test tubes in the sink. **Caution: test tubes may be hot!** If the tubes are hot, remove them using test tube tongs.

2. Clean the test tubes with a test tube brush.

3. Place test tubes in a test tube rack to dry.

Activity Questions

1. Describe the differences in color across the various concentrations of amylase.

   _____

   _____

2. Describe how enzyme concentration affected the amount of starch breakdown, or reaction rate.

   _____

   _____

   _____

   _____

3. If the 50% amylase solution and 10% amylase solution were allowed to sit for an hour in the test tube with the starch (before heating), do you think the results would have been different? Explain.

_____

_____

_____

4. Would the results have been different if the test tube with the 0% amylase solution were to sit for an hour before heat was applied? Explain.

_____

_____

_____

Post-Lab Assessment

Answer the following questions about the activities performed today.

1. Name the four organic compounds you tested.

   _____

   _____

2. A substance with a pH of 7.8 is:
   a. an acid
   b. a base

3. A substance with a pH of 3 is _____ times more acidic than a substance with a pH of 6.

4. A food scientist was testing the composition of a new food. She obtained a small sample of the food, put the food in a test tube, added a reagent, and then put the test tube in a water bath. One minute later, the food substance had turned bright red. What do these results indicate? What reagent was used?

   _____

   _____

   _____

5. Name the organic compound that amylase broke down. Name the product of amylase action.

   _____

   _____

6. Name the substance that contains the active site in the enzyme activity (Activity 3-3). Name the substance that is the substrate in the enzyme activity.

   _____

   _____

7. Two different enzyme properties were tested today. Name and describe both properties.

_____

_____

_____

8. **Critical Thinking:** The pH of urine fluctuates between 4 and 8, whereas the pH of blood is maintained between 7.35 and 7.45. Maintaining the homeostasis of acid/base balance in the blood is incredibly important for normal functioning. In fact, blood pH much higher than 7.5 or lower than 7.25 can result in death. Based on the fact that the acid/base balance of blood is so tightly regulated, why do you think that the pH of urine fluctuates so much?

_____

_____

_____

_____

_____

_____

_____

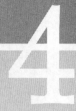

The Microscope

Textbook Correlation: Chapter 3—Cells and Tissues

Details

Activities	Activity Objectives	Required Materials	Estimated Time
4-1: Parts of a Microscope	Identify the parts of a microscope. Determine the magnification and total magnification of each lens	● Microscope	10–15 min
4-2: Focusing the Microscope	Focus the microscope under scanning as well as low and high powers	● Microscope ● Letter "e" slide	35 min
4-3: Microscope Properties: Depth Perception	Perceive depth using the microscope	● Microscope ● "Colored threads" slide	20 min
4-4: Preparing a Wet Mount	Prepare a wet mount	● Microscope ● Slide (clean and clear) ● Toothpicks ● Cover slip ● Methylene blue ● Biohazard container ● Bleach container ● Broken-glass container	15 min

Overview

Have you ever watched a TV show, such as *CSI*, and wondered what the forensic scientists were looking at under the microscope? Or how a microscope even works? Clinicians, pathologists, and forensic scientists use the microscope on a daily basis to observe many things, particularly cells and tissues. For example, a dermatologist may biopsy a suspicious-looking mole; that is, he or she will remove a small section of the mole and observe it under a microscope to examine the characteristics of the cells.

This laboratory exercise teaches you basic microscopy skills. We will be using the microscope throughout this course to observe all sorts of amazing cells and structures, such as sperm with flagellae, blood cells (erythrocytes and leukocytes), and nerve cells, just to name a few. So get the basics down today and you'll be ready to appreciate the beauty of different body cells later.

Need to Know

The microscope is made up of many parts, including the following:

- **Base:** The bottom of the microscope, which typically contains the on/off switch.

- **Stage:** A flat platform that holds the microscope slide, with the aid of **stage clips.**

- **Substage light:** The light located on the base of the microscope, which projects light up toward the stage.

- **Arm:** The angled, or bent, portion of the microscope to which the **ocular lens(es)** are attached.

- **Ocular lens(es):** The lens(es) that you look through in order to observe the specimen. There are two types of microscopes: uniocular scopes (one ocular lens) and binocular scopes (two ocular lenses). Many ocular lenses magnify the image (most by approximately 10 times).

- **Objective lens:** The lens that is closest to the specimen. There are typically four objective lenses that magnify at different levels (the amount of magnification varies by microscope brand). A lower magnification permits more of the specimen to be viewed; a higher magnification reveals more details of smaller structures. Generally, higher-magnification lenses are larger. In increasing order of magnification, the lenses are named:
  - **Scanning lens**
  - **Low-power lens**
  - **High-power lens**
  - **Oil-immersion lens** (This high-magnification lens requires you to place a small drop of oil on the slide in order to see the specimen clearly.)

- **Nose:** The structure that holds the objective lenses. You can rotate the nose in order to access the different objective lenses.

- **Coarse adjustment:** A large knob that moves the stage and objective lens closer to one another to bring the image into view.

- **Fine adjustment:** A smaller knob, usually projecting out from the coarse adjustment, that finely focuses on the image so that you can get a clear view.

- **Condenser:** A lens on the opposite side of the stage from the objective lens. It focuses the light hitting the stage and is typically adjusted when the high-power or oil-immersion lenses is in use.

- **Iris diaphragm lever:** A lever located below the stage that adjusts the intensity of the light hitting the stage.

Pre-Lab Activity

Students should complete this activity before completing the lab activities that follow.

Activity Instructions

Match the following definitions to the correct part of the microscope by writing the correct letter in the blank. Not all terms will be used and some terms may be used more than once.

Definitions

1. The objective lens that magnifies the least: _____

2. The largest knob, which brings the stage and objective lens closer together: _____

3. The flat horizontal section on which the slide (or specimen) is placed in order to view it: _____

4. The lens that you look through in order to view the specimen: _____

5. The lens located under the stage that focuses light onto the stage: _____

6. The lever that adjusts the intensity of the light that hits the stage: _____

7. The area of the microscope that holds the objective lenses: _____

8. The bottom of the microscope: _____

9. The types of objective lenses, listed in order of increasing magnification: _____

Microscope Parts

A. Arm
B. Base
C. Coarse adjustment
D. Condenser
E. Fine adjustment
F. High-power lens
G. Iris diaphragm lever
H. Low-power lens
I. Nose
J. Ocular lens
K. Oil-immersion lens
L. Scanning lens
M. Stage
N. Substage light

Parts of a Microscope

Activity Instructions

Identify the parts on your microscope. On the drawing below, write the correct part in each blank of the figure. The parts indicated with asterisks are not to be labeled on the figure.

Microsope Parts

- Base
- Stage
- Substage light
- Arm
- Ocular lens(es)
- Objective lenses
  - Scanning lens*
  - Low-power lens*
  - High-power lens*
  - Oil-immersion lens*

- Nose
- Coarse adjustment
- Fine adjustment
- Condenser
- Iris diaphragm lever*

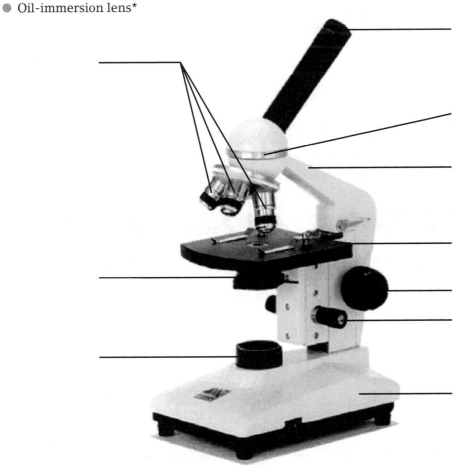

Activity Questions

1. Move the coarse adjustment knob while observing your microscope. Which part of the microscope moves: the stage or the nose?

_____

_____

2. Locate the knob that regulates the condenser. What happens to the condenser when you turn the knob?

_____

_____

3. Describe the difference in diameter between the coarse adjustment knob and the fine focus knob.

_____

_____

_____

4. Which objective lens in the shortest? The longest?

_____

5. As mentioned above, the objective lenses all magnify at various levels. The ocular lenses of many microscopes also magnify. The magnification of a lens is written on its barrel. For instance, the magnification of an oil-immersion lens is often 100×, which means that if the ocular lens magnifies 10×, the object viewed will be 1000 times larger than normal. Determine the magnification of each objective lens and the ocular lens (if any). Next, determine the total magnification by multiplying the magnification of the objective lens by that of the ocular lens. Fill in Table 4.1 with your answers.

Table 4.1 Magnification

Objective Lens	Objective Lens Magnification	Ocular Lens Magnification	Total Magnification
Scanning lens			
Low-power lens			
High-power lens			
Oil-immersion lens			

Focusing the Microscope

Activity Instructions and Questions

Follow the steps below to focus the microscope.

1. Plug in the microscope.

2. Ensure that the scanning lens (usually the smallest one) is facing the stage and that the **working distance** (distance between stage and objective lens) is at its maximum (stage and lens furthest apart).

3. Place the letter "e" slide on the stage (slide label facing you), securing the slide with the stage clips.

4. Move the slide so that the letter "e" is directly under the scanning lens.

5. Turn on the microscope.

6. Look through the ocular lens(es) and move the coarse adjustment knob until the image comes into view (the scanning lens is typically as close to the stage as possible). **Do not use coarse adjustment after this step!**

7. After the image is in the field of view, adjust with the fine focus knob until the image is clearly focused.

8. What did you observe regarding the position of the letter "e"? Draw your observations in the space below and use the lines provided to explain.

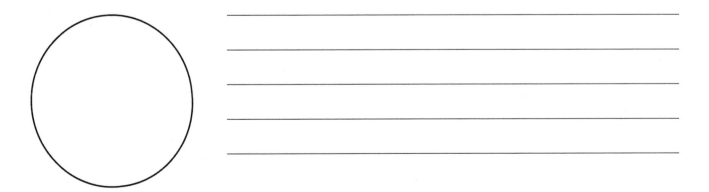

9. Increase the magnification to low power.

10. Use the fine focus adjustment knob to see the image clearly. Do not use the coarse adjustment knob during this step; if you do, start over on scanning power. Start over on scanning power if you cannot get the image in focus after adjusting fine focus.

11. Draw your observations in the space below. What happened to the **field size** (amount of object visible in the field of view) as the magnification increased from scanning power to low power? Why does the field size change? Explain, using the lines provided.

12. Increase the magnification to high power.

13. Use the fine focus adjustment knob to see the image clearly. Again, do not use coarse adjustment; if you do, start over on scanning power.

14. Draw your observations in the space below. What happened to the field size as you increased the magnification to high power? Why does the field size change? Explain, using the lines provided.

15. Adjust the condenser while on high power. Record your observations on the lines below.

16. Adjust the iris diaphragm lever while on high power. Record your observations on the lines below.

_____

_____

_____

17. To remove the slide, increase the working distance as much as possible using the coarse adjustment knob. Then move the revolving nose piece so that the scanning lens is facing the stage and release the slide from the slide clips.

You must stop and use fine focus at each lens. For example, if you wish to view an image under high power, you must first focus it under the scanning lens, then use fine focus on low power, and then again on high power. You cannot go directly from scanning power to high power without stopping at low power to tweak the fine focus.

Activity 4-3

Microscope Properties: Depth Perception

Activity Instructions

1. Obtain a colored threads slide and mount it on the stage.

2. Use the coarse adjustment to focus on the image; stay on scanning power.

3. Slowly turn the fine focus knob while looking at the threads. Do not look at the intersection of the threads but be sure to look somewhere in the field of view where all three threads are visible. Watch for the first thread in which the individual **fibers** of the thread are visible. That is the fiber that is on the top.

4. Repeat, this time looking for the thread that is in the middle.

5. Repeat again, looking for the thread that is on the bottom.

Activity Questions

1. Draw your observations in the space below and label the position of each thread on your drawing.

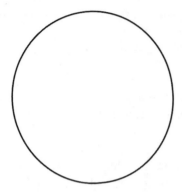

2. Which thread comes into clear focus first? The thread on the top, middle, or bottom?

_____

Activity 4-4

Preparing a Wet Mount of a Cheek Smear

A *wet mount* is a slide that suspends the specimen in liquid and uses a small piece of glass called a *cover slip* to keep the specimen in place. Today, you will prepare a cheek smear as an example of a wet mount. The term *wet mount* also refers to slides in which the specimen is a liquid, such as blood, urine, or semen.

Activity Instructions

Follow the instructions below to prepare a wet mount of a cheek smear.

1. Obtain a slide, toothpick, and cover slip.

2. Gently wipe the inside of your cheek with the toothpick and then spread the end of the toothpick that was in your mouth on a small center section of the slide.

3. Dispose of the toothpick in the biohazard pouch.

4. Place one or two drops of methylene blue on the center of the slide.

5. Cover that section of the slide with the cover slip.

6. Place the slide on the microscope and focus the slide under high power.

7. Draw your observations below.

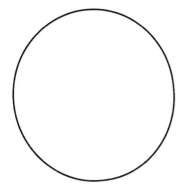

8. Cleanup: place the slide in a bleach container and dispose of the cover slip in a broken-glass container.

The flat, scalelike cells that you observed under the microscope are called **squamous epithelial** cells. The dark-staining center portion is the **nucleus** of the cell. The nucleus contains the DNA, which adheres to the dye, making it appear darker than the rest of the cell.

Activity Questions

1. What liquid was used to prepare the wet mount?

_____

2. Did you observe any other types of "cells" in your cheek smear? If you are taking an antibiotic, you might observe yeast in the oral cavity.

_____

Microscope Storage

Refer back to these instructions each time you use a microscope until performing the steps correctly has become second nature to you.

1. Turn off the microscope.

2. Increase the working distance as much as possible using the coarse adjustment knob.

3. Ensure that the scanning lens is facing the stage.

4. Remove the slide from the stage using the slide clips.

5. Adjust the condenser to its highest position (even with the stage).

6. Unplug the cord.

7. Coil and secure the cord.

Post-Lab Assessment

1. What is the total magnification of the high-power lens?

   _____

2. Which objective lens should be used first when you are focusing the microscope?

   _____

3. Which adjustment knob should NOT be used when you are observing a slide with the low-power lens?

   _____

4. What is the function of the condenser?

   _____

   _____

5. Define the term *working distance*.

   _____

   _____

5

Cell Anatomy and Life Cycle

Textbook Correlation: Chapter 3—Cells and Tissues

Details

Activities	Activity Objectives	Required Materials	Estimated Time
5-1: Cell Model Identification	Identify the components of a generalized cell	● Cell model	20 min
5-2: Cell Diversity	Investigate cellular diversity	● Microscope ● Slides (suggested: blood smear, teased smooth muscle, sperm, giant multipolar neuron)	25 min
5-3: Cell Life Cycle—Model	List and identify the stages of the cell life cycle List and identify the phases of the mitotic phase of the cell life cycle	● Play-Doh or other craft clay (multicolor set)	25 min
5-4: Cell Life Cycle—Microscope	Identify the phases of the cell life cycle on prepared slides	● Microscope ● Slides (suggested: whitefish blastocyte or onion)	25 min

Overview

Think of the city or town in which you live. Your town most likely has a mayor's office, a power plant, several factories, a shipping center such as the post office, and a waste removal service. All of these parts aid in the smooth running of your city or town. If one service stops, such as the power plant, most or all of the city or town is affected. Can you imagine if trash pickup services stopped in your neighborhood? Well, the human body contains trillions of little "cities" called cells. There are over 200 different types, all with different structures and functions. In this lab, you will observe four different types of cells found in the human body. All four look very different and have very different functions. And just as in a city, if services stop, the cell ceases to function. If many cells cease to function, the organ to which they belong may become diseased.

Need to Know

Cells are the basic structural and functional units of life.

- The cytoplasm contains the **cytosol**, or fluid portion of the cell, and the **organelles,** small structures that perform various cell functions.

- The organelles are similar to the parts of a city:
  - **Mitochondria**
    - ○ Produce energy in the form of ATP (similar to a power plant producing energy for a city)
  - **Ribosomes** and **rough endoplasmic reticulum**
    - ○ Synthesize proteins (factories)
  - **Golgi apparatus**
    - ○ Receives the proteins from the rough endoplasmic reticulum and packages them in vesicles for shipment (postal service)
  - **Lysosomes**
    - ○ Are Vesicles that break down old organelles or internalized wastes (trash service)
  - **Smooth endoplasmic reticulum**
    - ○ Performs various specialized functions, such as lipid synthesis, calcium storage, and detoxification (city offices)
  - **Nucleus**
    - ○ Contains information about the cell—the genetic code (in DNA) for making proteins (town hall)

- **Cytology** (the study of cells)
  - To visualize most organelles, specialized electron microscopes are required.
  - The nucleus, however, can be seen in any prepared slide; it is the dark-staining portion of the cell.

- Cells, much like us, have a life cycle. The two general phases of the life cycle are interphase and mitosis.
  - **Interphase**
    - The period between cell divisions.
    - Events include replicating DNA, making another centriole, and producing more cell organelles.
    - Many cells in adults are permanently in interphase and are not mitotically active.
  - **Mitosis** (nuclear division)
    - The division of the nucleus that results in two genetically identical nuclei.
      This consists of four phases:
        - **Prophase**
        - **Metaphase**
        - **Anaphase**
        - **Telophase**
  - **Cytokinesis**
    - The division of the entire cell into two identical daughter cells
    - Concludes the mitotic phase of the cell's life cycle

Pre-Lab Activity

Students should complete this activity before completing the lab activities that follow.

Activity Instructions

1. In the space below, draw a picture of a generalized cell, using Figure 3.4 in your textbook for reference.

2. Label all parts and organelles.

3. Using the lines provided, write a brief description of the function of each organelle. Be sure to explain it in scientific terms (e.g., not "powerhouse of the cell").

Cell Model Identification

Activity Instructions and Questions

1. On the cell model, identify the structures listed in the left-hand column of the table below. As you identify each structure, write down the corresponding number in the right-hand column.

Table 5.1   Cell Model Organelles

Cell Organelle	Number on Model
Cytosol	
Mitochondria	
Rough endoplasmic reticulum	
Smooth endoplasmic reticulum	
Golgi apparatus	
Centrioles	
Free ribosomes	
Fixed ribosomes	
Nucleus	
Nuclear membrane	
Nucleolus	

2. List similarities and differences in appearance between the rough endoplasmic reticulum and the smooth endoplasmic reticulum.

_____

_____

_____

3. Differentiate between the nucleus and nucleolus in terms of location and size.

_____

_____

_____

4. What is chromatin?

_____

5. Recall Laboratory 4, The Microscope. What do you think is the only part of the cell that is visible under the microscope? (Hint: Think of the cheek cell wet mount preparation.)

_____

Activity 5-2

Cell Diversity

Activity Instructions

1. Obtain one of each of the following slides and view at the magnification in parentheses:
   - Blood smear (high power)
   - Teased smooth muscle (low power)
   - Sperm (high power)
   - Giant multipolar neuron (high power)

2. Look at each slide under the microscope. Draw a picture in the circles below of what you see. Be sure to label the picture with the name of the slide and the magnification at which the drawing was made.

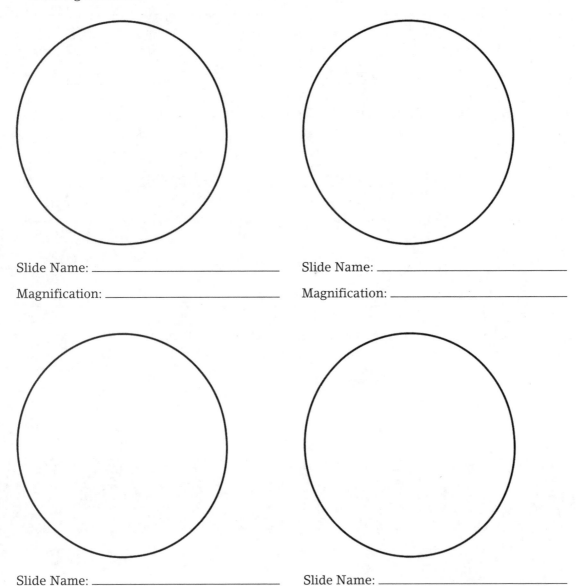

Slide Name: _____   Slide Name: _____

Magnification: _____   Magnification: _____

Slide Name: _____   Slide Name: _____

Magnification: _____   Magnification: _____

Activity Questions

1. What cell membrane modification does the sperm contain? Does any other human cell contain that modification?

_____

_____

2. Recall from Lab 4, The Microscope, that the nucleus stains darker than the rest of the cell, reflecting the presence of DNA. Was a nucleus present in most of the cells visible in the blood smear? (Note: these cells are the **erythrocytes,** or red blood cells.)

_____

_____

3. How is the structure of the neuron different from that of other cells? How do you think that the structure of the neuron relates to its function?

_____

_____

_____

_____

4. Describe the shape of the smooth muscle cells.

_____

_____

Activity 5-3

Cell Life Cycle—Model

Activity Instructions and Questions

Use the craft clay to construct the phases of the cell's life cycle.

1. Grab a handful of clay and roll it into a ball (about 2 or 3 inches in diameter). Continue rolling the ball in your hands to warm it up so it's more malleable.

2. Flatten the ball into a pancake. This is the cell.

3. With a different color of clay, make a ring to represent the nuclear envelope and place it in the center of the "cell."

4. Get a third color of clay. Roll it into a very thin long strand. Coil it up and place it in the nucleus. This is the chromatin.

5. A fourth color of clay will represent the centrosome. Mold the clay into a barrel shape and place it above the nucleus. What phase of the cell's life cycle is represented by the model you have created? What indicates that the "cell" is in that phase of its life cycle? Explain, using the lines below.

_____

_____

_____

6. Using more clay, create another "cell."

7. Use small pieces of clay with spaces between the pieces in order to represent the nuclear envelope as it disappears.

8. Get another color of clay and role it into several long thin strands. Place these in the nucleus. In this phase what is the arrangement of DNA called? How many of the thin strands representing the DNA should have been made in order to represent a real cell? Explain, using the lines below.

_____

_____

_____

9. Make two centrosomes and place them at opposite poles (sides) of the cell. This model represents early prophase.

10. Make a new cell.

11. Get another color of clay and make two sister chromatids. Join them together with a centromere and place it toward the center of the cell. How many pairs of sister chromatids should be in the cell?

_____

12. Make two centrosomes and place them at opposite poles (sides) of the cell. This represents late prophase.

13. Make a new cell.

14. Place the joined sister chromatids lined up in the middle of the cell (equatorial plane) and place the centrosomes at opposite ends of the cell. What phase of mitosis does it represent?

_____

_____

15. Make a new cell, but make it slightly longer than it is wide.

16. Make the sister chromatids again (now called chromosomes), but this time do not join them. Place them as if they were moving to opposite ends of the cell.

17. Place the centrosomes at opposite ends of the cell. This is anaphase.

18. Using the same cell, pinch the middle of the cell in so that it resembles an hourglass. What phase of the cell cycle is now represented? What is the purpose of this phase?

_____

_____

19. Read the description of telophase in your text and make a model to resemble that phase.

20. What phase of its life cycle does the cell go into after it completes telophase?

_____

21. As we can see from the models you made, a nucleus is required for a cell to enter mitosis. What other organelle is required?

_____

_____

22. Differentiate between mitosis and cytokinesis.

_____

_____

_____

Activity 5-4

Cell Life Cycle—Microscope

Activity Instructions

1. Obtain a slide that shows the stages of mitosis (whitefish blastula or allium root tip) and focus it under high power.

2. Look for the various stages of the cell's life cycle and draw an example of each in the circles below. Be sure to label the stage of the cell's life cycle and the magnification.
   - Interphase
   - Mitotic phase
     - Prophase
     - Metaphase
     - Anaphase
     - Cytokinesis

Life Cycle Stage: _____

Magnification: _____

Life Cycle Stage: _____

Magnification: _____

Life Cycle Stage: _____

Magnification: _____

Life Cycle Stage: _____

Magnification: _____

Activity Questions

1. In what phase of their life cycle are most of the cells?

   _____

2. Describe what each phase of mitosis looks like under the microscope.

   _____

   _____

   _____

   _____

   _____

   _____

   _____

Post-Lab Assessment

1. List the phases of the cell's life cycle.

_____

2. List the phases of mitosis in order.

_____

3. Name the phase of mitosis in which the chromatids are lined up along the equatorial plane.

_____

4. Name the structure that disappears during prophase.

_____

5. Critical Thinking: Why do you think that chromatin condenses into chromosomes before mitosis occurs?

_____

_____

_____

_____

_____

_____

_____

6. Write the name of the organelle next to the brief description of its structure.

    a. Contains an inner membrane folded into cristae: _____

    b. Interconnected network of membranes that is coated with ribosomes: _____

    c. Stack of membranes with hollow spaces: _____

    d. Tiny granules dispersed in the cytosol that can be located on another organelle and that synthesize protein: _____

    e. Interconnected network of membranes without any ribosomes on the surface: _____

    f. Resembles a barrel or "bundle of sticks": _____

6

Cell Membrane Transport and Permeability

Textbook Correlation: Chapter 3—Cells and Tissues

Details

Activities*	Activity Objectives	Required Materials (per group of 3–4 students)	Estimated Time
6-1: Effect of Tonicity on Osmosis	● Describe osmosis and its effect on tonicity ● Interpret data sets	● 4 potato discs (cut 1 inch thick) incubated for 2 or 3 hours in 0.3 M glucose solution ● Four 250-mL beakers ● Wax pencil ● Balance ● Distilled water ● Glucose solutions: 0.2 M, 0.4 M, 0.6 M	60–70 min
6-2: Selective Permeability and Diffusion	● Describe diffusion ● Describe how and why diffusion occurs ● Interpret data set	● 2 dialysis tubes (approx. 8 inches long) presoaked in 0.9% saline for at least 20 min ● 4 twist ties ● 10% glucose solution ● 2 graduated cylinders ● 2 funnels ● Three 250-mL beakers ● Wax pencil ● 10% starch solution ● Hot plate ● Test tube rack ● 4 test tubes ● 4 disposable transfer pipettes ● Benedict's reagent ● Iodine ● Test tube clamp	60 min

Details *(Continued)*

Activities*	Activity Objectives	Required Materials (per group of 3–4 students)	Estimated Time
6-3: Filtration	● Describe filtration ● Interpret data set	● Ring stand ● Funnel ● 250-mL beaker ● Filter paper ● Suspension (methylene blue, starch, coffee grounds)	10 min

*Note that activities 1 and 2 include long incubation times, during which other activities can be performed.

Overview

In this lab you'll be learning about osmosis, diffusion, and filtration, three mechanisms by which substances cross the cell membrane. Let's begin by looking at a familiar example of each.

Dominick and Bradley, 8-year-old best friends, love going outside after it rains, when snails come out of hiding. The boys always meet up with salt shakers in hand, find snails, and sprinkle them with salt. The salt-sprinkled snails shrivel up because of **osmosis,** which is the movement of water. Water follows salt, so the salt on the snail's surface draws water out of the snail's cells, causing it to shrivel. Today you will demonstrate osmosis by using potatoes incubated in glucose solutions. The solute concentration (osmolarity) of the solution surrounding the potato will cause the potato to gain or lose weight.

Have you ever been on a crowded elevator in a hotel? As soon as the doors open, the elevator crowd disperses into the lobby area, meeting up with friends, getting a cup of coffee, or heading to breakfast, the registration desk, or the front door. This scenario is a great example of diffusion (the movement of a solute from a high to a low concentration). The people in the elevator (high concentration) move to different areas of the lobby (low concentration) once the elevator doors open. Today's lab activities investigate both the practice and theory of diffusion.

Many people make coffee first thing in the morning. But what exactly is coffee? Coffee is the **filtrate** that forms when hydrostatic pressure forces water through coffee grounds and the pores in the coffee filter. Hydrostatic pressure forces hot water up a tube from the "tank" into the filter-lined coffee basket. The water molecules are small enough to pass through the pores of the filter and end up in the coffee pot; coffee grounds, however, are too large, so they remain in the filter basket. The end product is a filtrate of coffee-flavored water, or coffee! The most efficient filtration system in our bodies is in a special bed of capillaries, called the glomerulus, found in the kidneys. Today, you'll conduct an experiment to demonstrate filtration.

Need to Know

- ● **Osmosis**
  - ● The movement of water from an area of high concentration (low solute concentration) to an area of low concentration (high solute concentration)
  - ● **Osmolarity:** the total number of solutes in solution
  - ● Solutions containing **nonpenetrating solutes** (which cannot cross the cell membrane) cause changes in cell volume
    - ○ **Isotonic solutions** contain the same concentration of nonpenetrating solutes as the cytosol. There is no net movement in or out of the cell, so cell volume does not change. For example, a 0.9% (w/v) salt solution is isotonic with the cytosol and will not alter blood cell volume. It can safely be administered to increase blood volume.
    - ○ **Hypertonic solutions** contain a higher concentration of nonpenetrating solutes than the cytosol. Water leaves the cell; the cell then shrinks (crenates) and may die. For example, a 1.2% salt solution is hypertonic with the cytosol, so it will cause blood cells to shrink.
    - ○ **Hypotonic solutions** contain fewer nonpenetrating solutes than the cytosol. Water enters the cell; the cell then expands and may explode (lyse). For example, placing red blood cells in distilled water causes them to explode.

- ● **Diffusion**
  - ● The movement of a solute from an area of high concentration to an area of low concentration (down the concentration gradient)
  - ● **Simple diffusion**
    - ○ Penetrating solutes (lipids and gases) diffuse through the phospholipid bilayer.
    - ○ This process does not require any "assistance" from membrane proteins.
  - ● **Facilitated diffusion**
    - ○ Nonpenetrating solutes use membrane proteins to cross the cell membrane.
    - ○ There are two types of membrane proteins that assist in facilitated diffusion: **channels,** which form watery tunnels through the cell membrane for ions to cross, and **carriers,** which change shape to move specific solutes across the cell membrane.

- ● **Filtration**
  - ● Filtration is the movement of solutions through pores in a membrane.
  - ● The resulting collection of water and solutes is termed the **filtrate.**
  - ● The driving force of filtration is hydrostatic pressure.
  - ● Solute movement depends on the relative size of the particle and the pore.
    - ○ If the particle is smaller than the size of the pore, the particle will move and become part of the filtrate.
    - ○ If the particle is larger than the size of the pore, the particle will get "stuck" in the pore, will not move through, and will not become part of the filtrate.

Pre-Lab Activity

Students should complete this activity before completing the lab activities that follow.

1. When the salt dissolved in the water on the snail's skin, did it result in a hypertonic, isotonic, or hypotonic solution? What was the effect on the snail?

_____

_____

_____

_____

2. If you placed a cell in a hypotonic solution, what do you think would eventually happen?

_____

3. Based on the description of filtration in the overview, do you think that protein is part of the filtrate in a healthy individual? Explain your answer.

_____

_____

_____

_____

Activity 6-1

Effect of Tonicity on Osmosis

In this lab, you will investigate osmosis in potato cells. Water will move from a hypotonic solution into the potato cells, increasing the potato's mass. A hypertonic solution will cause the opposite effect.

Activity Instructions: Experimental Setup

Work in groups of 3 or 4 students. Read the following directions and then delegate the setup tasks.

1. Obtain 4 potato discs from the 0.3 M glucose solution and four 250-mL beakers and bring them back to your work station. Thoroughly dry the potato discs.

2. Label the beakers 1 through 4 with a wax pencil.

3. Weigh one potato disc and record the mass in Table 6.1.

4. Place the weighed potato disc in beaker 1.

5. Weigh potato disc 2, record its mass in Table 6.1, and place it in beaker 2.

6. Repeat this procedure for potato discs 3 and 4.

7. Fill beaker 1 with enough distilled water to submerge and cover the potato disc.

8. Fill beaker 2 with 0.2 M glucose solution; beaker 3 with 0.4 M glucose solution; and beaker 4 with 0.6 M glucose solution. Fill each beaker with enough solution to submerge the potato discs.

9. Allow the potato discs to incubate in the solutions for 45 to 60 minutes. You can complete some of the other lab activities while you wait.

Table 6.1 Potato Mass Data				
Potato/Beaker	Molarity of Solution	Mass Before (g)	Mass After (g)	Percent Change in Mass
1	0 M			
2	0.2 M			
3	0.4 M			
4	0.6 M			

Activity Instructions: Data Collection

1. Dry each potato disc thoroughly.

2. Weigh each potato disc individually and record the corresponding data in Table 6.1.

3. Calculate the percent change in mass of each potato disc, indicating a positive or negative percent change. The change in mass represents the amount of water lost or gained by the potato cells. Record in Table 6.1.

$$\text{Percent change (\%)} = [(\text{mass after} - \text{mass before}) / \text{mass before}] \times 100$$

Activity Instructions: Cleanup

1. Throw the potatoes away.

2. Pour the solutions down the drain.

3. Clean the beakers.

4. Return the rest of the supplies.

Activity Questions

1. Based on your data, which solutions were hypotonic? How do you know? What was happening to the potato cells placed in the hypotonic solution(s)?

_____

_____

_____

_____

2. Based on your data, which solutions were hypertonic? How do you know? What was happening to the potato cells placed in the hypotonic solution(s)?

_____

_____

_____

3. Were any of the solutions isotonic to the potato cells? If not, predict the concentration of glucose that would lead to an isotonic solution based on your data. Explain your answer.

_____

_____

_____

Selective Permeability and Diffusion

This lab compares the ability of two substances—large starch molecules and smaller glucose molecules—to diffuse across a membrane. We will use dialysis tubing, an artificial membrane, to simulate the cell membrane. Then, we will use Benedict's reagent to measure glucose diffusion out of the tubing and iodine to measure starch diffusion.

Activity Instructions: Experimental Setup

1. Obtain a dialysis tube and open both ends (best done by massaging the ends under running water).

2. Close off one end of the dialysis tube (twist ties work well).

3. Pour approximately 10 mL of 10% glucose solution into a 25-mL graduated cylinder.

4. Obtain a funnel and place the stem portion of the funnel into the open end of the dialysis tube.

5. Transfer the 10% glucose solution to the dialysis tube by pouring the contents from the graduated cylinder into the funnel.

6. Close the other end of the dialysis tube (twist ties work well).

7. Place the dialysis tube in a 250-mL beaker.

8. Use a wax pencil to label the beaker "G" (for glucose solution).

9. Pour enough water (tap water is fine) into the beaker to submerge the dialysis tube.

10. Obtain another dialysis tube and follow steps 1 and 2 above.

11. Pour approximately 10 mL of the 10% starch solution into a different 25-mL graduated cylinder.

12. Obtain a different funnel and place the stem of the funnel into the open end of the dialysis tube.

13. Transfer the 10% starch solution into the dialysis tube by pouring the contents from the graduated cylinder into the funnel.

14. Follow steps 6 and 7 above.

15. Use a wax pencil to label the beaker "S" (for starch solution).

16. Pour enough water (tap water is fine) into the beaker to submerge the dialysis tube.

17. Allow the dialysis tubes to incubate in the beakers for approximately 45 minutes.

Activity Instructions: Data Collection

1. Fill a 250-mL beaker approximately half full with tap water.

2. Place on a hot plate and turn on.

3. While waiting for the water to boil, obtain 2 test tubes from the test tube rack.

4. Using the wax pencil, label one test tube "DG" (for glucose solution from the dialysis tube) and the other "BG" (for glucose solution from the beaker) and place the test tubes back in the rack.

5. Remove the dialysis tube (with the glucose solution) from beaker "G" and open one end.

6. Obtain a sample of the fluid from the dialysis tube using a disposable transfer pipette.

7. Put the sample in the test tube labeled "DG" and place the test tube back in the rack.

8. Using a different disposable transfer pipette, obtain a sample of the fluid from beaker "G" and transfer the sample to test tube "BG."

9. Put several drops of Benedict's reagent in both test tubes.

10. Place the test tubes in the boiling water bath.

11. Observe for a color change and record your results in Table 6.2. If glucose is present, the solution will change from blue to green, yellow, orange, or red.

12. Turn off the hot plate and let the water and test tubes cool.

13. Obtain 2 different test tubes from the test tube rack and, using a wax pencil, label one "DS" (for the starch solution from the dialysis tube) and the other "BS" (for the starch solution from the beaker).

14. Use a third disposable transfer pipette and obtain a sample from the dialysis tube in beaker "S."

15. Transfer the sample to test tube "DS" and place in the test tube rack.

16. Repeat the above procedure to obtain a fluid sample from beaker "S" and place the sample in test tube "BS."

17. Put several drops of iodine in test tubes "DS" and "BS." Note that you do not need to use boiling water for this test.

18. Record the color of each sample in Table 6.2. If starch is present, the solution will change from brown to purple or black.

Table 6.2   Diffusion Data

Test Tube	Fluid Sample	Reagent Added	Color After Reagent Added*	Positive (+)/Negative (–) Result[†]
DG	Dialysis tube with glucose	Benedict's reagent		
BG	Beaker with glucose	Benedict's reagent		
DS	Dialysis tube with starch	Iodine		
BS	Beaker with starch	Iodine		

*Refer to Laboratory 3, Table 3.1 (Reagent Information) for a refresher as to how to interpret your color changes and data.
[†]Remember, a positive result indicates that the substance tested for is present (for instance, if glucose had a color change in test tube DG, that indicates a positive result, since it proved that glucose is present). If no color change occurs, that is a negative result, meaning that the substance tested for was not present.

Activity Instructions: Cleanup

1. Pour the contents of the test tubes, beakers, and dialysis tubes down the drain. (Note: use the test tube clamps if the test tubes are still hot.)

2. Rinse all glassware.

3. Throw away the dialysis tubes and disposable transfer pipettes.

4. Place the glassware, hot plate, twist ties, and test tube rack back where you found them.

Activity Questions

1. Based on your data, which substance (glucose or starch) diffused? How do you know? Fully explain your answer, supporting it with the data you obtained.

_____

_____

_____

_____

_____

_____

2. Why do the data make sense? (Hint: Think about the organic molecules described in Chapter 2.)

_____

_____

_____

_____

3. The dialysis tube's pores were large enough to allow one substance to diffuse from it and into the surrounding beaker water by simple diffusion. Can that substance utilize simple diffusion when moving in and out of our cells? Explain your answer.

_____

_____

_____

Filtration

This activity examines the filtration of three substances of different sizes—coffee grounds, starch, and methylene blue.

Activity Instructions: Experimental Setup

1. Get a ring stand, funnel, 250-mL beaker, filter paper, and container of suspension (contains methylene blue, coffee grounds, and starch).

2. Place the funnel in the ring on the ring stand and place the beaker below the funnel (to collect the **filtrate**).

3. Lightly dampen the filter paper with deionized water.

4. Fold the filter paper into a cone and place it in the funnel.

5. Shake the suspension well until all of the components are well mixed.

6. Slowly pour approximately 10 mL (just eyeball it) of suspension into the filter paper–lined funnel.

7. Wait a few minutes before proceeding to the data collection section.

Activity Instructions: Data Collection

1. Look at the filter paper and in the filtrate for the presence of coffee grounds. Put a check mark in Table 6.3 in the place(s) in which the coffee grounds are visible.

2. Look at the filter paper and in the filtrate for the presence of methylene blue (a blue liquid). Put a check mark in the table below in the place(s) in which the methylene blue is visible.

3. Put several drops of iodine both in the beaker and on the filter paper. Watch for a color change indicating the presence of starch. Put a check mark in the table below in the place(s) in which there is a positive test result for starch.

Table 6.3 Filtration Data

Suspension Component	Presence in Filter Paper	Presence in Filtrate
Coffee grounds		
Starch		
Methylene blue		

Activity Instructions: Cleanup

1. Pour the contents of the beaker down the drain and rinse the beaker.

2. Throw away the filter paper.

3. Place all items back where you found them.

Activity Questions

1. Which substance(s) is/are part of the filtrate? Explain the results referring to the data table.

_____

_____

_____

2. Explain why not all of the substances became part of the filtrate.

_____

_____

_____

_____

3. **Critical Thinking:** Which organ in the body is our major "filtration" system? What liquid does it filter? Why is the liquid filtered? What does the filtrate become?

_____

_____

_____

_____

_____

Post-Lab Assessment

1. **Critical Thinking:** In the past few years, many college fraternities have gotten into big trouble for hazing during pledge week. One such hazing technique that has received national attention is induced water toxicity, in which the pledge is forced to consume copious amounts of water. This has led to the death of some pledges. Based on what you now know regarding tonicity, did the blood plasma become hypertonic or hypotonic? Explain. What do you think led to these deaths?

_____

_____

_____

_____

_____

2. **Critical Thinking:** Glomerulonephritis is an inflammatory condition of the kidneys that increases the capillary permeability of the glomeruli (capillary beds in the kidneys). One result is proteinuria, or protein present in the urine. How can the protein become part of the filtrate in this disease?

_____

_____

_____

_____

7
Histology

Textbook Correlation: Chapter 3—Cells and Tissues

Details

Activities	Activity Objectives	Required Materials	Estimated Time
7-1: Identifying Epithelial Tissue	Identify various types of epithelial tissue	● Colored pencils ● Microscope ● Epithelial tissue slides (see Instructor Resources for some ideas)	60–70 min
7-2: Identifying Connective Tissue	● Identify various types of connective tissue ● List the components of connective tissue ● Identify cells and fibers in various types of connective tissue	● Colored pencils ● Microscope ● Connective tissue slides (see Instructor Resources for some ideas)	60–70 min
7-3: Mystery Slides	Apply knowledge gained in the previous laboratory exercises	● Colored pencils ● Microscope ● Organ slides (see Instructor Resources for some ideas)	10–20 min

Overview

Just after her 14th birthday, Shavani went for her annual checkup. Her physician recommended that she undergo yearly **Pap smears** to screen for cervical cancer. In this simple procedure, the physician obtains a cell sample from the **cervix,** which is the opening to the uterus. The cells are smeared on a glass slide and examined microscopically. Any questionable results are sent to a **pathologist**, who specializes in the analysis of tissue for the presence of disease. Shavani agreed to the test, and one week later her physician asked her to come back to discuss the results. The physician began, "Shavani, we detected an abnormality in your Pap smear. Some of the cells look distinctly different from normal cells, and we are a bit concerned that these abnormal cells might develop into cancer." To be on the safe side, Shavani underwent laser surgery, which eradicated the abnormal cervical cells. Happily, a follow-up Pap smear 6 months later did not show any abnormalities.

Cervical cancer can be deadly because it often causes symptoms only after it spreads to other tissues. Many lives are saved by the early diagnosis of cervical precancerous growths using Pap smears. The ability to recognize healthy and unhealthy tissue is thus a critical skill for all health professionals. Today's lab introduces **histology,** the study of tissue. We concentrate on two types of tissue: epithelial tissue and connective tissue.

Remember that histology requires practice and patience. If you take the time to precisely focus your microscope and really *look* at the slides, you will see amazing details emerge from what initially appears to be a "sea of pink." The more time that you invest in learning to recognize the types of epithelial and connective tissues, the easier it will be in future labs when you revisit these tissues as components of specific organs.

Need to Know

- **Epithelial tissue**
  - Consists of tightly packed cells joined together by tight junctions.
  - Lines the **lumen** (or interior space) of hollow organs and makes up the top layer (epidermis) of the skin. The **basal** surface of the epithelium rests on a dense protein mat called the **basement membrane.** The **apical** surface of the epithelium lines the lumen and may have modifications, such as cilia or microvilli.
  - It is classified by the number of cell layers:
    - **Simple** epithelium consists of a single layer of cells, which all attach to the basement membrane.
    - **Stratified** epithelium consists of two or more layers of cells, and only one layer attaches to the basement membrane.
  - Also classified by cell shape:
    - **Squamous** cells are flat (resembling fish scales).
    - **Cuboidal** cells are boxy, with large central nuclei.
    - **Columnar** cells are tall, with nuclei close to the basement membrane.
  - Example: *simple cuboidal epithelium* is a single layer of box-shaped cells.

- **Connective tissue**
  - Develops from primitive embryonic tissue called **mesenchyme.**
  - Consists of cells separated by the **extracellular matrix.**
    - ○ Cells include fibroblasts or specialized cells.
    - ○ Extracellular matrix consists of protein fibers suspended in a featureless gel called **ground substance.**
    - ○ Ground substance can be liquid (such as blood plasma), gel-like, or even solid (as in bone).
  - Example: blood
    - ○ Blood cells are erythrocytes and leukocytes.
    - ○ Blood has a ground substance called **plasma,** which contains water, protein, glucose, and electrolytes.
    - ○ Fibers (fibrinogen) are present in blood only during injury.
  - Example: dense connective tissue proper
    - ○ Its cells are fibroblasts.
    - ○ It has minimal ground substance.
    - ○ It has collagen protein fibers.

Pre-Lab Activity

Students should complete this activity before completing the lab activities that follow.

1. Describe the difference in the number of cell layers between simple epithelium and stratified epithelium.

    _____

    _____

2. Comparing epithelial and connective tissues, which tissue type contains closely packed cells? Which tissue type contains cells further apart and also includes fibers?

    _____

    _____

    _____

    _____

Identifying Epithelial Tissue

This activity asks you to classify different epithelial tissues based on cell shape and the number of layers. See Figure 3.27 in your textbook for illustrations of the different types of epithelial tissue.

Activity Instructions

1. Look at slides containing epithelial tissue. Remember, you are looking for tightly packed cells (cells right next to one another). Note that one slide contains abnormal (cancerous) epithelial tissue.

2. Use colored pencils to draw what you see in the corresponding circles below. Add a written description to support your drawing. The drawings or descriptions should be good enough that you can study them at home and remember what the specific tissue looks like.

3. Label the drawings, record the total magnification (TM), and record the name of the slide. Most slides are best observed at either low or high power.

4. Look at several different slides showing the same type of tissue and record the names of those slides.

Simple Squamous Epithelium

TM _____

Slide name _____

Other slides _____

_____

Description _____

_____

_____

_____

_____

Simple Cuboidal Epithelium

TM _____

Slide name _____

Other slides _____

_____

Description _____

_____

_____

_____

_____

Simple Columnar Epithelium

● Look for **microvilli** on some slides.

● Look for **goblet cells** on some slides.

TM _____

Slide name _____

Other slides _____

_____

Description _____

_____

_____

_____

_____

Pseudostratified Columnar Epithelium

● Look for **cilia** on some of the slides.

● Look for **goblet cells** on some slides.

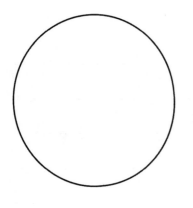

TM _____

Slide name _____

Other slides _____

_____

Description _____

_____

_____

_____

_____

_____

Nonkeratinized Stratified Squamous Epithelium

TM _____

Slide name _____

Other slides _____

_____

Description _____

_____

_____

_____

_____

Keratinized Stratified Squamous Epithelium

TM _____

Slide name _____

Other slides _____

_____

Description _____

_____

_____

_____

_____

Keratinized Stratified Squamous Epithelium (Cancer)

TM _____

Slide name _____

Description _____

_____

_____

Stratified Cuboidal Epithelium

TM _____

Slide name _____

Other slides _____

_____

Description _____

_____

_____

_____

_____

Stratified Columnar Epithelium

TM _____

Slide name _____

Other slides _____

_____

Description _____

_____

_____

_____

_____

Activity Questions

1. Describe the difference in appearance between keratinized and nonkeratinized stratified squamous epithelium.

   _____

   _____

   _____

2. Explain what the word *pseudostratified* in pseudostratified columnar epithelium refers to.

   _____

   _____

   _____

3. Describe the difference in the number of cell layers between stratified cuboidal epithelium and stratified squamous epithelium (keratinized or nonkeratinized).

   _____

   _____

   _____

4. Describe the general structure of epithelial tissue.

   _____

   _____

   _____

5. Describe the differences between the skin cancer slide (keratinized stratified squamous epithelium) and the normal skin slide.

   _____

   _____

   _____

Identifying Connective Tissue

This activity asks you to classify connective tissue based on the identity of the cells and the composition of the extracellular matrix. See Figure 3.30 in your textbook for images of the different types of connective tissue.

Activity Instructions

1. Look at slides containing connective tissue.

2. Use colored pencils to draw what you see in the corresponding circles below. Add a written description to support your drawing. The drawings or descriptions should be good enough that you can study them at home and remember what the specific tissue looks like.

3. Label the drawings, record the total magnification (TM), and record the name of the slide. Most slides are best observed at either low or high power.

4. Name the type(s) of cells and fiber(s) seen. Name the ground substance for each type of connective tissue, even if you cannot see it.

5. Look at several different slides showing the same type of tissue and record the names of those slides.

Mesenchyme

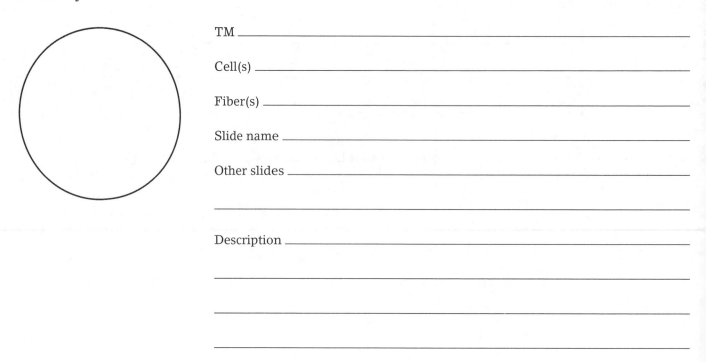

TM _____

Cell(s) _____

Fiber(s) _____

Slide name _____

Other slides _____

_____

Description _____

_____

_____

_____

Loose Areolar Tissue

TM _____

Cell(s) _____

Fiber(s) _____

Slide name _____

Other slides _____

_____

Description _____

_____

_____

_____

Adipose Tissue

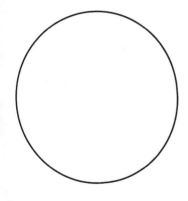

TM _____

Cell(s) _____

Fiber(s) _____

Slide name _____

Other slides _____

_____

Description _____

_____

_____

_____

Dense Connective Tissue

TM _____

Cell(s) _____

Fiber(s) _____

Slide name _____

Other slides _____

_____

Description _____

_____

_____

_____

Hyaline Cartilage

TM _____

Cell(s) _____

Fiber(s) _____

Slide name _____

Other slides _____

_____

Description _____

_____

_____

_____

Fibrocartilage

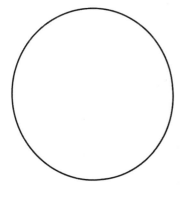

TM _____

Cell(s) _____

Fiber(s) _____

Slide name _____

Other slides _____

_____

Description _____

_____

_____

_____

Elastic Cartilage

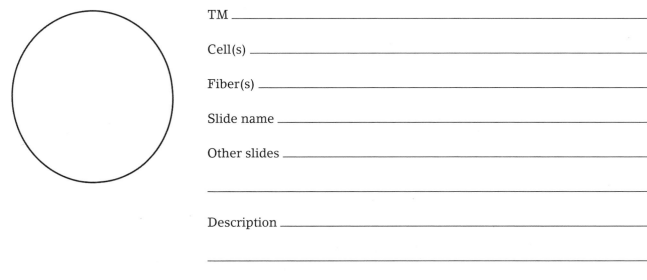

TM _____

Cell(s) _____

Fiber(s) _____

Slide name _____

Other slides _____

_____

Description _____

_____

_____

_____

Blood

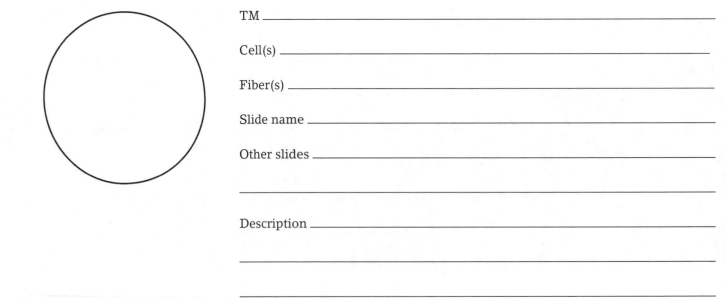

TM _____

Cell(s) _____

Fiber(s) _____

Slide name _____

Other slides _____

_____

Description _____

_____

_____

_____

_____

Bone Tissue

TM _____

Cell(s) _____

Fiber(s) _____

Slide name _____

Other slides _____

_____

Description _____

_____

_____

_____

Activity Questions

1. Adipocytes in adipose tissue look "empty" but are not. What is found in the adipocyte? Is the substance ever used? If so, when?

_____

_____

_____

2. Think about the structure of dense (fibrous) connective tissue. Why does it make sense that ligaments and tendons are composed of that specific tissue?

_____

_____

3. Describe the differences in appearance between the three types of cartilage.

_____

_____

_____

4. **Critical Thinking:** Epithelial tissue is avascular (does not contain blood vessels) but is alive, therefore requiring oxygen and glucose. How, exactly, does it receive nutrients? Through diffusion from underlying connective tissue! Review the connective tissues that you have seen under the microscope and the types of cells and extracellular matrix that each contains. Which one of these tissues do you think underlies most epithelial tissues? Support your answer with facts and observations. (Hint: The answer here is not "blood." The epithelium needs the gases from blood, however, so the tissue must be a type that is highly vascularized. "Adipose" is not the correct answer because adipose tissue typically surrounds the entire organ.)

_____

_____

_____

_____

_____

_____

_____

Mystery Slides

Activity Instructions

1. View the demonstration microscopes that have different slides and different total magnifications.

2. Use colored pencils to draw what you see in the corresponding circles. Add written descriptions to support your drawings. Determine the type of tissue for each slide. Record your answers below.

3. After recording all of your answers to the mystery slides, check your answers. For any missed identification, go back to the microscope and look at the slide again. Figure out the source of error and write down any new observations.

Mystery Slide 1

TM _____

Description _____

_____

_____

Tissue type _____

Mystery Slide 2

TM _____

Description _____

_____

_____

Tissue type _____

Mystery Slide 3

TM _____

Description _____

_____

_____

Tissue type _____

Mystery Slide 4

TM _____

Description _____

_____

_____

Tissue type _____

Post-Lab Assessment

1. Color each of the following figures according to the color key listed below:
   - Chondrocytes: green
   - Collagen fibers: pink
   - Columnar epithelium: gray
   - Cuboidal epithelium: orange
   - Elastic fibers: blue
   - Erythrocytes: red
   - Fibroblasts: brown
   - Leukocytes: purple
   - Osteocytes: yellow
   - Squamous epithelium: black

2. Write the name of each type of tissue beside or below the image.

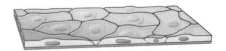

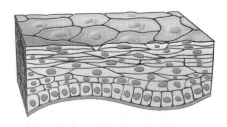

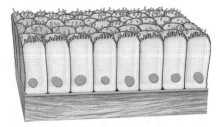

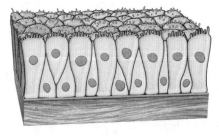

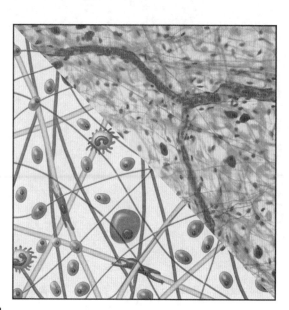

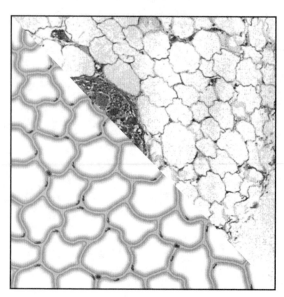

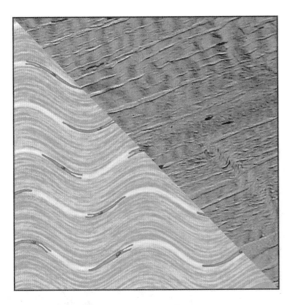

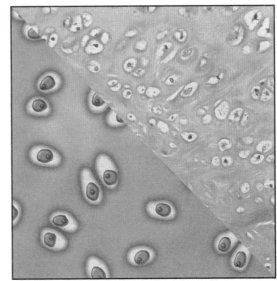

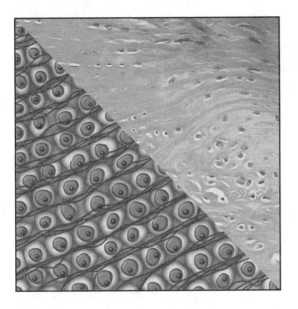

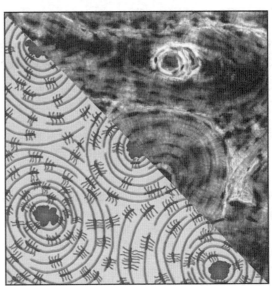

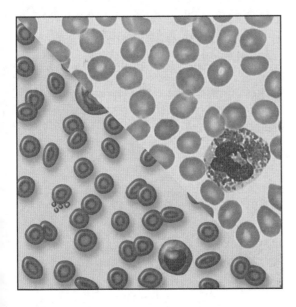

8

The Skin and Associated Structures

Textbook Correlation: Chapter 5—Skin, Membranes, and Other Barriers to the Environment

Details

Activities	Activity Objectives	Required Materials	Estimated Time
8-1: Identifying Parts of the Skin	Identify regions, layers, and accessory structures of the skin on models	● Skin model	25 min
8-2: Microscopic Anatomy of the Skin	Identify the regions, layers, and eccrine glands of the skin microscopically	● Microscope ● Skin slide ● Cancer slide	20 min
8-3: Microscopic Anatomy of Hairy Skin	Identify parts of hair and the structures associated with hair	● Microscope ● Hairy skin slide	20 min
8-4: Fingerprint Analysis	Analyze fingerprints	● Index cards (unruled) ● Ink pad	15 min
8-5: Nail Anatomy	Identify the parts of a nail	● Colored pencils	10 min

Overview

Remember Sylvester from the Chapter 5 case study? He died as a result of burns over a large area of his body. His head, neck, and arms received partial-thickness burns, whereas his torso suffered full-thickness burns. But what does this mean, and why are burns so harmful? In order to appreciate the critical importance of skin as the body's primary barrier to the environment, it is important to understand its structure. It is important to maintain the integrity of the skin in order to prevent dangerous pathogens, ultraviolet radiation, and other deadly things from entering the body. In today's lab, you will learn the parts of the intact skin and observe the skin's thickness and associated structures under the microscope.

Need to Know

The skin, or integument, is composed of two general regions:

- **Epidermis** is composed of five layers (strata)
  - **Stratum corneum:** the thickest layer (20-30 cell layers) of dead, keratinized epithelial cells.
  - **Stratum lucidum:** thin, translucent layer only present in the thick skin
  - **Stratum granulosum:** darkly staining cells containing protein granules
  - **Stratum spinosum:** multiple layers of plump cells that assume a spiny appearance in histological preparations
  - **Stratum basale:** single layer of stem cells
  - The deepest layer damaged in superficial thickness burns

- **Dermis** is composed of two layers
  - **The papillary** (superficial) **layer** comprises 20% of the dermis.
    - ○ Composed of areolar connective tissue
    - ○ Supplies the avascular epidermis with nutrients
    - ○ Contains upward projections called **dermal papillae,** which are responsible for fingerprints
    - ○ The deepest layer damaged in superficial partial-thickness burns
  - **The reticular layer** comprises 80% of the dermis
    - ○ Composed of dense connective tissue
    - ○ Contains randomly arranged collagen fibers that allow skin to stretch in many directions
    - ○ The deepest layer damaged in deep partial thickness burns

The **subcutaneous layer** is located below the skin.

- Composed of areolar connective tissue.

- Attaches skin to the underlying skeletal muscle.

- Provides nutrients to the skin.

- Absorbs shock and insulates the body.

- Full-thickness burns penetrate into the subcutaneous region and sometimes into underlying muscle and bone tissue.

Many accessory structures are contained in skin.

- **Hair** is composed of a soft keratinized epithelium.
  - **Follicle:** epithelial tissue sheath surrounding the hair
  - **Arrector pili:** band of smooth muscle that contracts to make the hair stand up

- Skin **glands** are exocrine glands (secrete onto body surface).
  - **Sebaceous glands** secrete sebum (oil) into the hair follicle in order to moisturize the skin and hair.
  - **Eccrine sudoriferous glands** secrete watery sweat through pores to the surface of the skin and are located throughout the body.
  - **Apocrine sudoriferous glands** secrete an oilier sweat and are associated with hair follicles in the armpits and groin.

- **Sensory receptors** in skin include:
  - Free nerve endings: detect pain and temperature
  - Meissner corpuscles: nerve ending surrounded by a few layers of epithelial tissue
  - Pacinian corpuscles: nerve ending surrounded by many layers of epithelial tissue

- **Nails** are a hard, keratinized epithelium used as a tool and for grooming.

Pre-Lab Activity

Students should complete this activity before completing the lab activities that follow.

Activity Instructions

Match the following terms with the correct definition. Not all terms will be used.

1. The most superficial region of the skin: _____

2. Primary (largest) layer of the dermis: _____

3. Structure that secretes oil (sebum) into the hair follicle: _____

4. Layer that is present only in thick skin, such as in the palms and soles: _____

5. Band of smooth muscle that is connected to the hair follicle: _____

6. Unique pattern of folds that project into the epidermis and are responsible for fingerprints: _____

7. Stem cell layer that is one cell thick: _____

8. Gland that secretes sweat into pores: _____

9. Layer of areolar connective tissue that is located below the skin: _____

A. Arrector pili
B. Dermal papillae
C. Dermis
D. Epidermis
E. Hair follicle
F. Papillary layer
G. Reticular layer
H. Sebaceous gland
I. Stratum basale
J. Stratum corneum
K. Stratum granulosum
L. Stratum lucidum
M. Stratum spinosum
N. Subcutaneous layer
O. Sudoriferous gland

Identifying Parts of the Skin

This activity will increase your familiarity with the parts of skin by requiring you to identify them on a model.

Activity Instructions

1. Obtain a skin model.

2. Locate the following structures on the model if your model has numbers, and fill in the corresponding number in Table 8-1.

Table 8.1 Skin Structure and Model Correlation			
Skin Structure	**Number on Model**	**Skin Structure**	**Number on Model**
Epidermis		Dermal papillae	
Dermis		Hair root	
Hypodermis (subcutaneous layer)		Hair follicle	
Stratum corneum		Hair shaft	
Stratum lucidum		Arrector pili	
Stratum granulosum		Sebaceous gland	
Stratum spinosum		Sudoriferous gland	
Stratum basale		Eccrine gland	
Papillary layer		Apocrine gland	
Reticular layer			

Activity Questions

1. In the table above, are the epidermal strata listed from superficial to deep or from deep to superficial?

   _____

2. Name the deep layer of the dermis.

   _____

3. Name the layer of the dermis that is in contact with the epidermis. Name the stratum of the epidermis that the dermal layer touches.

   _____

   _____

4. Name two structures associated with hair.

   _____

5. Name the duct through which the sebaceous gland secretes sebum (oil).

   _____

   _____

Microscopic Anatomy of the Skin

Activity Instructions

1. Obtain the palm slide and identify the structures listed below.

2. Draw and label your findings. Write a brief description of what you observe.

3. After looking at the palm slide, look at the skin cancer slide. You viewed the skin cancer slide in the tissue lab, but now you can see the disorganization of structure. Draw, label, and describe your findings.

Regions (scanning, low, and high powers)

- Epidermis
- Dermis

Layers (low and high powers)

- Stratum corneum
- Stratum lucidum
- Stratum granulosum
- Stratum spinosum
- Stratum basale

Accessory Structures (low and high powers)

- Eccrine gland
- Hypodermis

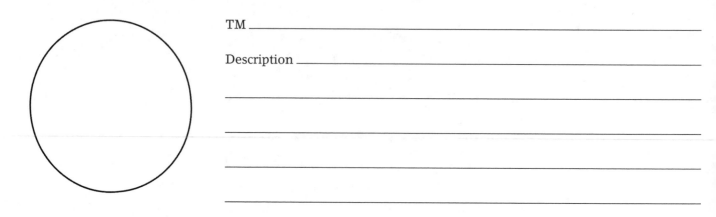

TM _____

Description _____

_____

_____

_____

_____

TM _____

Description _____

_____

_____

_____

_____

TM _____

Description _____

_____

_____

_____

_____

TM _____

Description _____

_____

_____

_____

_____

Activity Questions

1. Name the tissue that makes up the epidermis.

   _____

2. Name the tissue that makes up the papillary layer of the dermis.

   _____

3. Name the tissue that makes up the reticular layer of the dermis.

   _____

4. Name the tissue that makes up the eccrine gland.

   _____

5. Name the tissue that makes up the hypodermis.

   _____

6. Describe the differences observed between the healthy skin slide and the cancerous skin slide. Use the new terminology learned in this lab (regions, layers, tissue, structures).

   _____

   _____

   _____

   _____

   _____

   _____

Microscopic Anatomy of Hairy Skin

Activity Instructions

1. Obtain the hairy skin (scalp) slide and identify the structures listed below.

2. Draw and label your findings. Write a brief description of what you observe.

Regions (scanning, low, and high powers)

- Epidermis
- Dermis

Accessory Structures

- Hair (scanning, low, and high powers)
  - Hair root
  - Hair follicle
- Sebaceous gland (scanning, low, and high powers)
- Arrector pili (low and high powers)

TM _____

Description _____

_____

_____

_____

TM _____

Description _____

_____

_____

_____

TM _____

Description _____

_____

_____

_____

TM _____

Description _____

_____

_____

_____

Activity Questions

1. Name the general type of tissue that makes up the hair follicle and sebaceous gland.

_____

2. Describe the specific location of the hair root and sebaceous gland (region and layer).

_____

_____

3. Describe several differences between the thick skin (palm) and the scalp. Include layers and structures present in the different locations.

_____

_____

_____

_____

_____

Fingerprint Analysis

The unique pattern of the dermal papillae is obvious in very thin skin, such as the skin of the fingertips. Sweat from the eccrine sudoriferous glands coats these ridges. When a surface (such as glass) is touched, a characteristic pattern of sweat is deposited that can be visualized using forensic techniques. Several different patterns of fingerprints—such as loops, whorls, and arches—are shown in the figures below: (a) arch, (b) loop, and (c) whorl. This activity involves solving a burglary case using fingerprint evidence.

One dark stormy night, a burglar took advantage of a power outage and broke into the evidence room at the local police precinct. Fortunately the burglar was not able to steal anything because the power was quickly restored. The burglar did, however, leave behind fingerprints.

You and your classmates are the suspects, and you have been rounded up for fingerprint analysis. Two of you are actually police detectives and will quickly be cleared. The detectives will then take and analyze the fingerprints of the rest of the suspects until the burglar is found.

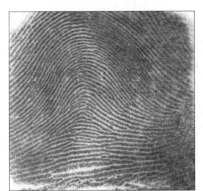

a. Arch

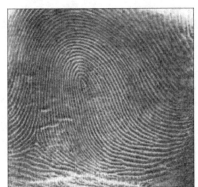

b. Loop

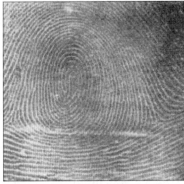

c. Whorl

Activity Instructions

1. Get an index card and an ink pad.

2. Write your name in pencil on the index card.

3. Turn the index card over so that your name cannot be seen.

4. Slowly and gently roll your right thumb over the ink from right to left.

5. Place your thumb on the left side of the index card and transfer your fingerprint by rolling the thumb from left to right.

6. Repeat the above instructions with your right index and middle fingers. Place the index finger print in the middle of the index card and the middle finger print on the right side of the index card.

7. Give your index card to your instructor.

8. Once the instructor has received an index card from each student in the class, the instructor will randomly choose three index cards. The instructor will announce two names from the three chosen index cards. Those two students are the "detectives." The other student, whose name is not announced, is the "burglar." The rest of the class, including the burglar, are suspects.

9. The instructor provides the crime scene evidence (fingerprints of the "burglar") to the detectives.

10. The two detectives take the suspects' fingerprints by following steps 1 through 6 above. The "cleared" suspects (whose fingerprints do not match the "burglar's") help the detectives analyze the fingerprints.

11. Stop once the burglar has been apprehended.

Activity Questions

1. Identify the pattern of your fingerprints.

_____

_____

2. Did some of the suspects have similar fingerprints? If so, how did you conclude which was the burglar?

_____

_____

_____

3. What was the most common fingerprint pattern?

_____

_____

Nail Anatomy

Activity Instructions and Questions

1. In the space below, draw your finger (including the nail) and label the following parts of the nail using a different color pencil for each structure. Use Figure 5.17 of the textbook if required.

- Proximal nail fold
- Eponychium
- Lunula
- Lateral nail fold
- Nail
- Free edge

2. Draw a midsagittal section of the finger and nail and label the following parts with a different color pencil for each structure.

- Nail matrix
- Eponychium
- Lunula
- Nail plate
- Hyponychium
- Bone (phalanx)
- Dermis
- Epidermis

Post-Lab Assessment

1. On the figure below, color each skin layer according to the following key:

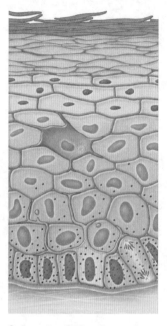

- Dermis: brown
- Stratum basale: yellow
- Stratum corneum: green
- Stratum granulosum: purple
- Stratum lucidum: orange
- Stratum spinosum: blue

2. Color the following structures using the color key below. Note: Some structures may appear more than once, so color all locations for each structure.

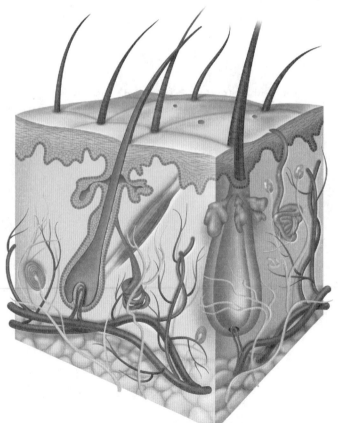

- Arrector pili: red
- Dermis: brown
- Eccrine gland: purple
- Epidermis: blue
- Hair follicle: brown
- Hair root: green
- Hair shaft: black
- Sebaceous gland: orange
- Subcutaneous region: yellow

3. Areolar connective tissue contains many blood vessels. Why does it make sense that the papillary layer of the dermis is composed of areolar connective tissue?

_____

_____

_____

4. List the general fingerprint patterns.

_____

_____

5. Determine whether the following statement is true. If it is false, explain why. "The hypodermis is considered a true region of the skin."

_____

_____

_____

9

Introduction to Bones and Joints

Textbook Correlation: Chapter 6—Bones and Joints

Details

Activities	Activity Objectives	Required Materials	Estimated Time
9-1: Bone Model	Label the parts of a long bone.	● Bone Model	15 min
9-2: Microscopic Anatomy of Compact Bone	Observe and identify the parts of compact bone microscopically.	● Compact bone slide ● Microscope ● Chicken bone incubated in vinegar (1–2 days) ● Chicken bone incubated in proteolytic enzymes	15 min
9-3: Bone Markings	Identify a variety of bone markings on several bones.	● 3 Skulls ● 2 Vertebrae ● Femur (thigh bone) ● 2 Os coaxae (hip bones) ● Humerus ● Mandible (jawbone) ● Midsagittal skull ● 3 blue pipe cleaners ● 3 yellow stickers ● 1 pink pipe cleaner ● 3 green stickers ● 3 red stickers ● 1 blue sticker ● 2 orange stickers	45 min
9-4: Movements at Synovial Joints: "Simon Says"	Define and perform the different movements at synovial joints.	● No materials required	15–20 min

Details *(Continued)*

Activities	Activity Objectives	Required Materials	Estimated Time
9-5: Types of Synovial Joints	Give examples of the different types of synovial joints.	• Articulated skeleton	45 min
9-6: The Parts of a Synovial Joint: Knee Joint Anatomy	Label the parts of a synovial joint.	• Knee joint model • Optional: Raw chicken wings and dissection equipment	15–25 min

Overview

Imagine the following scenario: Riding your bike down a steep hill, you run into a post and soar over the handlebars, landing on your outstretched right arm. Chances are you will have injured one or more organs of your skeletal system—bones. X-rays would reveal the bones beneath the injured skin and show various bone features, or markings, that might be useful for localizing the sites of your bone fractures.

If your injured upper limb were placed in a full-length cast, you would suddenly become aware of another important part of your skeletal system—the joints. Joints (also called articulations) permit one bone to move in relation to another, so using the injured arm for most activities (such as scratching an itchy nose) would be impossible. Joint movements can be described in relation to the joint involved or to the moving bone. Thus, this movement could be described as elbow flexion or forearm flexion.

Today's lab explores the basic structures of the skeletal system—bones and joints. In particular, we will focus on the structure of bone tissue as well as the structure and function of a specific type of joint called the synovial joint.

Need to Know

Bone, as you may remember from the tissue lab, is a type of connective tissue. It is derived from embryonic mesenchyme and contains an extracellular matrix and cells. The extracellular matrix is composed of osteoid, collagen, and mineralized salts. The cells found in bone are the osteoblasts, osteoclasts, and osteocytes. Only osteocytes will be visible in today's lab. Two types of bone tissue exist, compact bone and spongy bone, each with a very different structure and function.

Bone Terminology

- **Osteons:** cylindrically shaped components of **compact bone**
  - **Lamellae:** rings of mineral and collagen fibers that make up an osteon
    - ○ Look like the rings of a tree stump
  - **Central canals:** spaces that run vertically in each osteon
    - ○ Blood vessels, lymphatic vessels, and nerves run through the space
  - **Osteocytes:** cells that are interspersed between the lamellae
    - ○ **Lacuna:** a space in which the osteocytes are located

- **Perforating canals:** spaces that radiate horizontally from the central canal and carry blood vessels and nerves, connecting to various central canals
- **Canaliculi:** Small passageways containing osteocyte processes through which solutes pass

- **Trabeculae:** networks of **spongy bone**
  - Replace osteons
  - Contain lamellae
  - Arrangement is not concentric, as it is in compact bone
    ○ Blood vessels pass through the trabeculae rather than in a central canal

- **Long-bone regions:**
  - **Diaphysis:** bone shaft (long axis of bone)
    ○ Primarily composed of compact bone
    ○ Has a thin internal layer of spongy bone
    ○ **Medullary cavity:** space in the center of the diaphysis
  - **Epiphyses:** proximal and distal ends of bone
    ○ Outer, thin layer of compact bone
    ○ Primarily composed of internal spongy bone
    ○ No medullary cavity
  - **Metaphysis:** region between the diaphysis and the epiphysis

- **Membranes:**
  - **Periosteum:** surrounds all of the diaphysis and most of the epiphyses
    ○ Made of dense connective tissue
  - **Endosteum:** thin membrane that lines the medullary cavity
  - **Articular cartilage:** surrounds a small portion of the epiphyses
    ○ Made of hyaline cartilage
    ○ Prevents the end of the bone from rubbing with the articulating bone

Movements at Synovial Joints

(Note that all movements are in reference to the anatomical position.)

- **Flexion:** decreasing the angle between the two bones
- **Extension:** increasing the angle between the bones, usually back toward the anatomical position
- **Abduction:** moving the body part further away from the midline of the body
- **Adduction:** bringing the body part closer to the midline of the body
- **Protraction:** moving one bone anteriorly
- **Retraction:** moving one bone posteriorly
- **Elevation:** moving one bone superiorly
- **Depression:** moving one bone inferiorly
- **Circumduction:** tracing a circle with the moving body part
- **Rotation:** pivoting one bone around its axis
- **Gliding:** moving two bones with flat articulating surfaces past one another
- **Plantarflexion:** standing on your tiptoes
- **Dorsiflexion:** standing on your heels
- **Inversion:** moving the soles of the feet toward one another
- **Eversion:** moving the soles of the feet away from one another
- **Pronation:** moving the palms posteriorly
- **Supination:** moving the palms anteriorly

Types of Synovial Joints

● **Gliding:** consists of two flat articulating surfaces in which one bone smoothly moves (glides) past the other
  ● Can move in many directions but is typically limited in range

● **Pivot:** occurs when one bone rotates around another bone
  ● Allows for pronation and supination
  ● Example: the radius pivots (rotates) around the ulna

● **Hinge:** evident when one articulating surface is curved in a U or C shape and articulates with an indented structure.
  ● Allows for flexion and extension
  ● Example: the elbow

● **Condyloid:** concave (rounded indention in the middle) surface articulates with a convex (rounded projection in the middle) surface
  ● Allows for two planes of motion
  ● Example: the joints between the fingers and palm
  ● Allows for both:
    ○ Finger abduction/adduction
    ○ Finger flexion/extension

● **Saddle:** resembles two perpendicular saddle structures articulating together
  ● Example: the thumb

● **Ball-and-socket:** round head of one bone fits into a cup-shaped depression in the second articulating bone
  ● Allows for a large range of motion
  ● Example: the shoulder

Pre-Lab Activity

Students should complete this activity before completing the lab activities that follow.

1. Label the following drawing using the terms listed below:
   - Central canal
   - Compact bone
   - Lamellae
   - Medullary cavity
   - Osteocyte
   - Perforating canal
   - Periosteum
   - Spongy bone

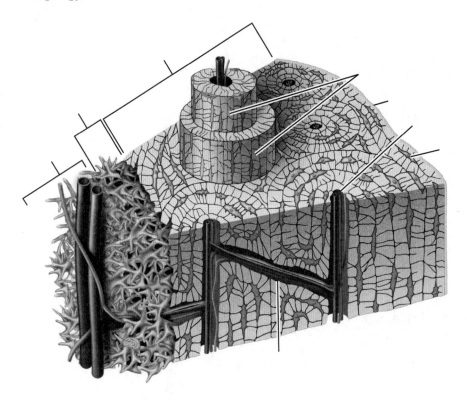

2. Draw arrows indicating movement on the following illustrations.

   a. Draw an arrow on the image below indicating flexion of the thigh.

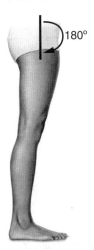

180°

   b. Draw an arrow on the image below indicating abduction of the thigh.

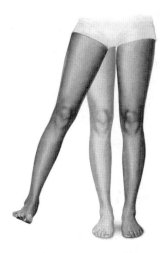

   c. Draw an arrow on the image below indicating plantarflexion.

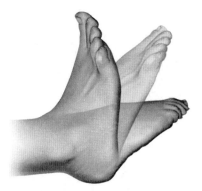

Bone Model

Activity Instructions

On the bone model, identify the structures listed in the left-hand column of Table 9-1. As you identify each structure, write down the corresponding number in the right-hand column.

Table 9.1 Bone Model	
Structure	**Number**
Periosteum	
Osteon	
Central canal	
Perforating canal	
Lamellae	
Osteocytes	
Lacunae	
Canaliculi	
Trabeculae	
Red marrow	

Activity Questions

1. Describe the difference between the lacuna and the lamella.

_____

_____

_____

2. Describe the differences in structure between compact bone and spongy bone.

_____

_____

_____

Activity 9-2

Microscopic Anatomy of Compact Bone

Activity Instructions

1. Obtain a compact bone slide and observe it under low and high powers. Identify the parts: central canal, lamellae, osteocytes, canaliculi.

2. Draw, label, and describe your findings and then answer Activity Questions 1 and 2 below.

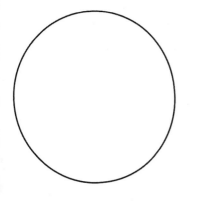

TM _____

Slide name _____

Description _____

_____

_____

_____

TM _____

Slide name _____

Description _____

_____

_____

_____

_____

3. Microscopic Anatomy Demonstration

   a. Two chicken leg bones were incubated in two different solutions. One chicken bone has been incubated in vinegar (acetic acid) for 1 to 2 days and the other was incubated in proteolytic enzymes (enzymes that break down protein).

   b. Put on gloves and remove the bones from the labeled containers. Gently blot each bone with a paper towel. Touch each bone and answer Activity Questions 3 and 4 below.

Activity Questions

1. Name the structure that forms the rings around the central canal.

   _____

2. Name the cells that you observed under the microscope.

   _____

3. How does the bone incubated in vinegar feel? Recalling that vinegar (acetic acid) is a weak acid, what do you think happened to the chemical constituents of bone tissue? Hint: Think about the acids stored in osteoclasts as well as the function of osteoclasts.

   _____

   _____

   _____

   _____

4. Compare the texture/consistency of the bone incubated in the proteolytic enzymes with that of the bone incubated in vinegar. What do you think happened to the chemical constituents of the bone tissue?

_____

_____

_____

_____

Activity 9-3

Bone Markings

Activity Instructions and Questions

Bones contain many markings, which have a wide variety of functions—such as muscle attachment, bone articulation, or providing a passageway for blood vessels. The bones listed below have been marked to show various bone markings:

- Mandible (jawbone)
- Skull
- Midsagittal skull
- Vertebrae (backbone)
- Femur (thigh bone, the longest bone in the body)
- Pelvis
- Humerus (arm bone)

Some bones may have been marked to show more than one bone marking. Each bone marking is color-coded (for example, all of the fossae are indicated with a yellow sticker). The color of each bone marking is listed after the name of the bone marking.

1. **Foramina** (sing., foramen) have been indicated with blue pipe cleaners. Observe the blue pipe cleaner on the skull, vertebra, and pelvis. How would you describe this bone marking?

_____

_____

2. **Fossa** (yellow sticker). Observe the yellow stickers on the skull and humerus. Based on your observations, what is a fossa?

_____

_____

_____

3. **Fissure:** (pink pipe cleaner). A pink pipe cleaner can be located on the skull. How would you describe a fissure? How does it differ from a foramen?

_____

_____

_____

4. **Condyle** (green sticker). Look for the green stickers on the mandible (jawbone), the skull, and the femur (thigh bone). How would you describe a condyle?

_____

_____

_____

5. **Process** (red sticker). Look for three red stickers on a vertebra (part of the backbone). What is a process?

_____

_____

_____

6. **Tuberosity** (blue sticker). The blue sticker is on the pelvis. How would you describe a tuberosity?

_____

_____

_____

7. **Sinus** (orange sticker). The midsagittal skull contains two orange stickers. What is a sinus, based on your observations?

_____

_____

_____

Movements at Synovial Joints: "Simon Says"

Activity Instructions

This is the joint version of the classic childhood game. The instructor will play the part of "Simon" and will instruct students to demonstrate the various types of synovial joint movements. For example, the instructor may state "Simon says flex the forearm" and you would flex at the elbow joint. Remember, do the movements only when the instructor first says "Simon says"! Keep in mind the difference between the arm and forearm as well as the thigh and leg. You can get more information about movements at each joint in the illustrations at the end of Chapter 7.

Activity Questions

1. In which movement is the joint angle between the thigh and leg decreased?

2. Which movement brings the arm closer to the midline of the body?

3. Which movement are you doing when you stand on your tiptoes?

4. What movement are you doing when you stand on the lateral (outside) surfaces of your feet?

5. What positions are your arms in when you are standing in standard anatomical position? List as many as you can.

Types of Synovial Joints

Activity Instructions

1. Find each joint illustrated in the figure on an articulated skeleton. Using the articulated skeleton model, manipulate each joint, but keep in mind that your joints do not have the same degree of motion because of the presence of skeletal muscle and connective tissue.

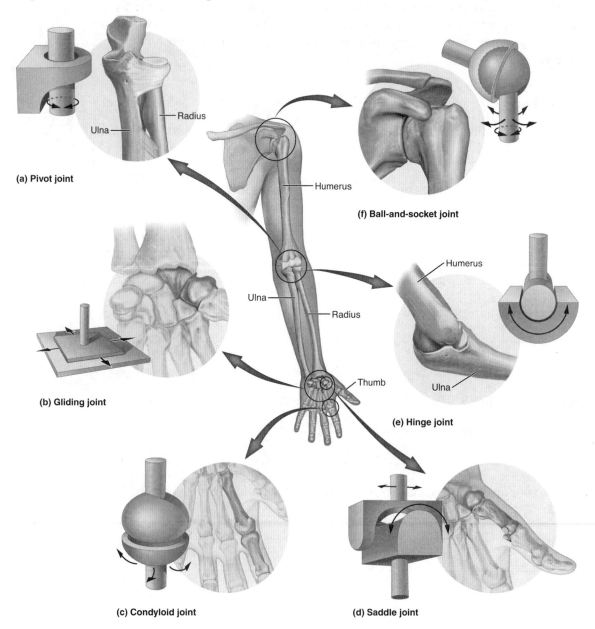

(a) Pivot joint

Radius
Ulna
Humerus

(f) Ball-and-socket joint

(b) Gliding joint

Ulna
Radius
Thumb

Humerus

(e) Hinge joint

Ulna

(c) Condyloid joint

(d) Saddle joint

2. Now perform the same movement with your own body parts.

Activity Questions

1. Which movements allowed for a fairly similar degree of movement between the skeleton and your body? Explain, citing specific examples.

_____

_____

_____

_____

2. Which movements allowed for a very different degree of movement between the skeleton and your body? Explain, citing specific examples.

_____

_____

_____

_____

3. **Critical Thinking:** Look at the articulating surfaces of the two ball-and-socket joints in the body. One of the joints is more prone to injury owing to the structure of the articulating surfaces. Which ball-and-socket joint do you think is more prone to injury? Why?

_____

_____

_____

_____

The Parts of a Synovial Joint: Knee Joint Anatomy

Activity Instructions

See page 219 of the textbook for more information about the structure of the knee joint.

On the knee joint model, identify the structures listed in the left-hand column of Table 9.2. As you identify each structure, write down the corresponding number in the right-hand column.

Table 9.2 Knee Joint Model	
Structure	**Number on Model**
Tendon of quadriceps muscle	
Bursa	
Anterior cruciate ligament	
Posterior cruciate ligament	
Tibial collateral ligament	
Fibular collateral ligament	
Meniscus	

Activity Questions

1. Describe the structural and functional differences between a tendon and a bursa.

_____

_____

_____

_____

_____

2. **Critical Thinking:** Which is more likely to damage the knee joint: a blow to the lateral aspect of the joint or a blow to the popliteal area? Explain your answer.

_____

_____

_____

_____

_____

_____

Knee Joint Dissection (Optional)

Activity Instructions

1. Put on gloves and obtain a raw chicken wing.*

2. Place the chicken wing on a dissecting tray. Use your scalpel to remove the skin and muscle from the bones. Be careful around the joint between the upper and lower wing so that you do not sever the ligaments and tendons in the area.

3. Observe the joint capsule, articulating surfaces, ligaments, and tendons of the chicken wing.

4. Wash your hands with warm water and soap and sanitize your work space.

5. Draw and label your findings below.

***CAUTION: Raw poultry can carry *Salmonella*. Avoid contacting your face, eyes, and ears with your hands while working with the raw chicken and afterwards until you have removed your gloves and properly sanitized your hands at the end of the activity.**

Activity Questions

1. What joint in your body is homologous to the joint between the upper and lower wing of the chicken?

   _____

2. How do the articulating surfaces appear similar between the human and the chicken? How do the surfaces appear different?

   _____

   _____

   _____

Post-Lab Assessment

1. Name the shaft of a long bone.

   _____

2. Name the membrane that surrounds the shaft of the bone.

   _____

3. Name the small passageways containing osteocyte processes through which solutes pass.

   _____

4. What is the name of a rounded hole in a bone?

   _____

5. What is the name of a hollow cavity in the skull?

   _____

6. Name the movement that juts the jaw forward.

   _____

7. Name the movement that occurs when you stand on your heels.

   _____

8. Name the structural classification of the most movable synovial joint.

   _____

9. What is the name of a tissue structure that connects bone to bone?

   _____

10

Axial Skeleton

Textbook Correlation: Chapter 6—Bones and Joints

Details

Activities	Activity Objectives	Required Materials	Estimated Time
10-1: Cranial Bones and Bone Markings	Identify the bones and bone markings of the cranium; identify the hyoid bone.	● Skull ● Disarticulated cranial bones ● Hyoid bone ● Fetal skull ● Colored pencils	50 min
10-2: Facial Bones and Bone Markings	Identify the bones and bone markings of the face.	● Skull ● Disarticulated facial bones	30 min
10-3: Build and Draw a Skull	Identify the articulations between the different cranial and facial bones.	● Disarticulated skull bones ● Colored pencils	15 min
10-4: Vertebral Column Bones and Bone Markings	Identify the bones and bone markings of the vertebral column.	● Articulated vertebral column ● Disarticulated vertebral column ● Colored pencils	30 min
10-5: Sternum and Rib Bones and Bone Markings	Identify the bones and bone markings that make up the thoracic cavity.	● Articulated skeleton ● Ribs ● Sternum ● Colored pencils	15 min

Overview

Every day, more than 100 Americans die in motor vehicle accidents. Many of these deaths could be prevented if drivers and passengers always wore seat belts. During one such fatal accident, the driver, a healthy 19-year-old male, broke several of the thoracic vertebrae surrounding the delicate spinal cord. Surgeons were able to remove the bone fragments, preventing them from penetrating the spinal cord. In the same accident, the passenger was not so lucky. He was thrown from the car, fracturing his skull and first two cervical vertebrae. This resulted in traumatic brain injury and transection of the cervical spinal cord, and he died at the scene.

Most of the bones in the axial division protect delicate organs. The skull protects the brain, the vertebrae protect the spinal cord, and the thoracic cage protects the heart and lungs. In today's lab you will use models and drawing activities in order to learn the bones and bone markings of the axial skeleton.

Need to Know

- The skull consists of the:
  - **Cranium,** the bony enclosure of the brain
  - **Facial bones,** which form the skeletal structure of the face
  In the table below, the number in brackets indicates whether the bone is paired (2) or unpaired (1).

Cranial Bones	Facial Bones
Frontal bone (1)	Maxillary bone (2)
Parietal bone (2)	Palatine bone (2)
Occipital bone (1)	Zygomatic bone (2)
Temporal bone (2)	Lacrimal bone (2)
Sphenoid (1)	Vomer (1)
Ethmoid (1)	Nasal bone (2)
	Mandible (1)

- The **hyoid:**
  - U-shaped bone.
  - One of the few freely floating bones in the body, meaning that it does not articulate with any other bone.

- The **vertebral column** is divided into five structurally and functionally distinct regions:
  - **Cervical** vertebrae:
    - There are 7.
    - Their small size allows for the greatest range of motion of all of the vertebral regions.
    - The **atlas (C1)** and **axis (C2)** are first two cervical vertebrae; they are most unique in appearance and allow the head to pivot.
  - **Thoracic** vertebrae:
    - There are 12.
    - They are characterized by long spinous processes.
    - The ribs articulate with the thoracic vertebrae.
  - **Lumbar** vertebrae:
    - There are 5.
    - They are large and sturdy.
    - They receive most of the load when one is bending over, lifting heavy objects, and sitting.
  - **Sacrum:**
    - Begins as five different bones and eventually fuses into one bone in the adult.
    - Contains many foramina for the passage of spinal nerves.
  - **Coccyx:**
    - Most inferior vertebral bone.
    - Fuses from 5 bones to form 2 to 4 bones in the adult skeleton.
    - This is what breaks when a person breaks the "tailbone."

- **Sternum** and **ribs:**
  - Form the thoracic cavity
  - Sternum—flat bone divided into three regions:
    - The superior **manubrium.**
    - The **body.**
    - A small process called the **xiphoid process.** Avoidance of the xiphoid process is very important in giving CPR. If too much pressure is applied to the xiphoid process, it can break off and puncture the liver.
  - The ribs:
    - Articulate with the thoracic vertebrae posteriorly and with the sternum anteriorly.
    - There are 12 pairs.
    - Classified according to the articulation with the sternum: "true ribs," "false ribs," and "floating ribs."
      - First 7 pairs of ribs are true ribs and have a direct costal cartilage connection to the sternum.
      - False ribs connect to the costal cartilage of the seventh rib.
      - The two floating ribs do not connect to cartilage.

Pre-Lab Activity

Students should complete this activity before completing the lab activities that follow.

1. Define *foramen*.

_____

_____

2. Name the cranial bones and specify which are paired and which are unpaired.

_____

_____

_____

_____

3. Name the facial bones and specify which are paired and which are unpaired.

_____

_____

_____

_____

4. List the regions of the vertebral column from superior to inferior. As you do, list the number of
   bones that make up each vertebral region both during embryonic growth and in the adult.

_____

_____

_____

_____

Cranial Bones and Bone Markings

Activity Instructions

On the articulated and disarticulated skull, identify the bones and bone markings listed in the left-hand column of Table 10.1. As you identify each bone and bone marking, write a description in the right-hand column. See Figures 6.20 to 6.27 (and accompanying narrative) of the textbook for information about the different bones.

Table 10.1 Cranial Bones	
Bone or Bone Marking	**Description**
Parietal bones	
Temporal bones	
Zygomatic processes	
External auditory meatuses	
Styloid processes	
Mastoid processes	
Mandibular fossae	
Carotid canals	

Table 10.1 Cranial Bones (continued)

Bone or Bone Marking	Description
Jugular foramina	
Occipital bone	
Occipital condyles	
Foramen magnum	
Sphenoid bone	
Sphenoid sinus	
Sella turcica	
Foramina ovale	
Optic foramina	
Ethmoid bone	
Superior nasal conchae	
Middle nasal conchae	

(continued)

Table 10.1 Cranial Bones (continued)

Bone or Bone Marking	Description
Ethmoid sinuses (air cells)	
Cribriform plate	
Perpendicular plate	
Crista galli	
Frontal bone	
Frontal sinus	
Fetal skull fontanels: anterior, posterior, anterolateral	
Frontal, coronal, sagittal, lambdoid, squamous sutures	
Hyoid bone (not part of cranium)	

Activity Questions

1. Color the temporal bone blue and label the following bone markings on the figures below:
   - Zygomatic process
   - External auditory meatus
   - Mastoid process
   - Styloid process
   - Mandibular fossa
   - Carotid canal

2. Color the occipital bone red and label the following bone markings on the figures below:
   - Foramen magnum
   - Occipital condyles

3. Color the ethmoid bone purple and label the following bone markings on the figures below:
   - Cribriform plates
   - Crista galli
   - Perpendicular plate

4. Color the sphenoid bone green and label the following bone markings on the figures below:
   - Sella turcica
   - Foramen ovale
   - Optic foramen
   - Sphenoid sinus

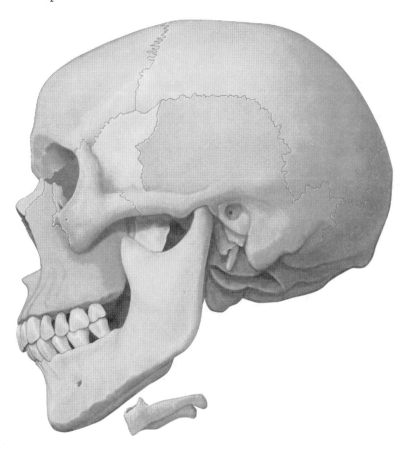
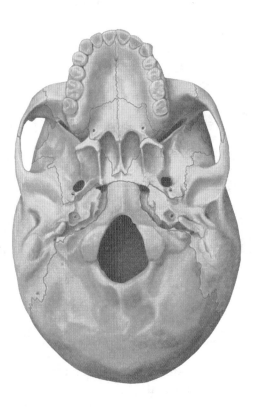

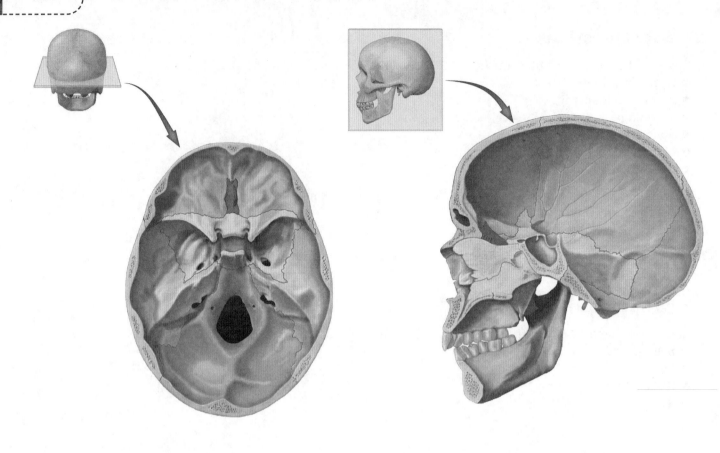

Activity 10-2

Facial Bones and Bone Markings

Activity Instructions

On the articulated and disarticulated skull, identify the bones and bone markings in the left-hand column in Table 10.2. As you identify each bone and bone marking, write a description of it in the right-hand column. See Figures 6.20, 6.21, 6.23, 6.24, and 6.27 (and accompanying narrative) in your textbook for more information.

Table 10.2　Facial Bones

Bone or Bone Marking	Description
Maxillae	
Alveolar margin	
Maxillary sinuses	
Palatine processes (hard palate)	
Palatine bones	
Zygomatic bones	
Lacrimal bones	
Lacrimal ducts	
Mandible	
Mandibular condyles	
Alveolar margin	
Vomer	
Nasal bones	

Build and Draw a Skull

Activity Instructions

1. Use the disarticulated cranial and facial bones to build your own skull. Take particular note of the articulations between the different skull bones.

2. The following illustrations show the bones of the face and skull but without any lines dividing the bones.
   a. Draw lines separating the different skull bones on the figures below.
   b. Find the sphenoid in each view and color it the same color. Color the circle next to the word *sphenoid* using this same color.
   c. Repeat step b for the other bones, using different colors.

   ○ Frontal bone   ○ Occipital bone
   ○ Ethmoid   ○ Lacrimal bones
   ○ Sphenoid   ○ Vomer
   ○ Mandible   ○ Temporal bones
   ○ Maxillae   ○ Zygomatic bones
   ○ Parietal bone   ○ Nasal bones

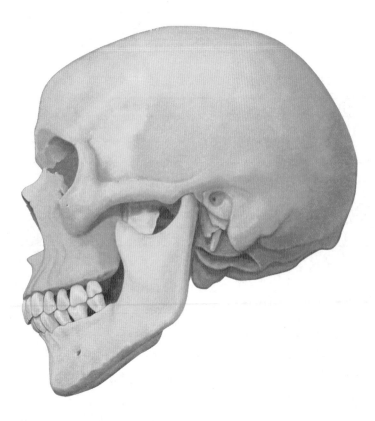
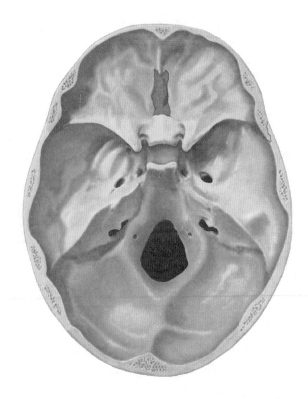

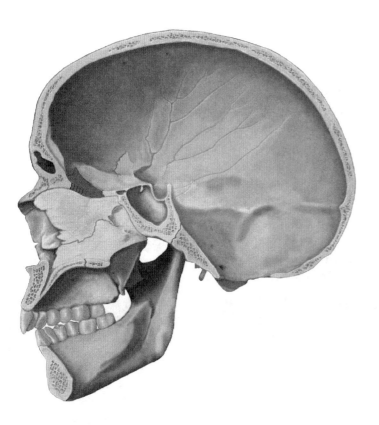
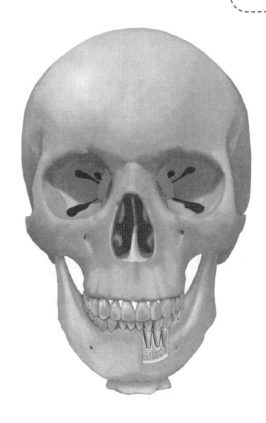

Activity Questions

1. Name two bones that articulate with the zygomatic bone.

_____

2. Name two different bones that embed the roots of teeth.

_____

3. Name the bones that form the eye orbit.

_____

4. Name the bones that form the nasal cavity.

_____

5. If someone smacked you in the back of the head, what bone would they hit?

_____

Vertebral Column Bones and Bone Markings

Activity Instructions

On the articulated and disarticulated vertebral column models, identify the characteristic or bones listed in the left-hand column of Tables 10.3 and 10.4. As you identify the characteristic or bone, write down a description in the right-hand column. See Figures 6.28 and 6.29 (and accompanying narrative) of the textbook for more information.

Table 10.3   General Vertebral Characteristics

Characteristic (Bone Marking)	Description
Body	
Vertebral arch	
Pedicles	
Laminae	
Vertebral foramen	
Spinous process	
Transverse process	
Superior articular processes	
Inferior articular processes	
Intervertebral foramen	

Table 10.4 Vertebrae	
Bone or Bone Marking	**Description**
Atlas (C1)	
Anterior arch (instead of body)	
Axis (C2)	
Dens (odontoid process)	
Cervical vertebra	
Transverse foramina	
Thoracic vertebra	
Lumbar vertebra	
Sacrum	
Sacral canal	
Sacral hiatus	
Sacral foramina	
Coccyx	

Activity Questions

1. Articulate several thoracic vertebrae and use them to answer questions 1 through 3. Describe how the bones articulate with one another by identifying the specific articulating processes.

_____

_____

_____

2. Name the hole that goes down the center of the articulated vertebrae. Name the structure that is located in the hole.

_____

3. Name the hole that is found between the transverse processes of the articulated vertebrae. What do you think passes through those holes?

_____

4. Color the following structures, using the color key, on the illustrations below.
   - Pedicle: red
   - Lamina: orange
   - Body: blue
   - Transverse process: green
   - Spinous process: purple
   - Superior articular process: brown
   - Inferior articular process: yellow

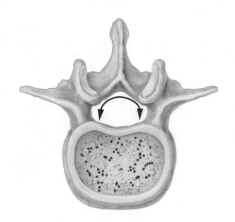   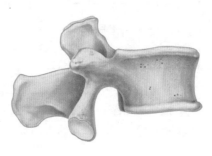

Sternum and Ribs and Bone Markings

Activity Instructions

On the articulated and disarticulated skeleton, identify the bones and bone markings listed in the left-hand column of Table 10.5. As you identify the bone and bone markings, write a description in the right-hand column. See Figure 6.31 of the textbook.

Table 10.5 Sternum and Ribs	
Bone or Bone Marking	**Description**
Sternum	
Manubrium	
Clavicular notch	
Suprasternal (jugular) notch	
Sternal angle	
Body	
Xiphoid process	
Ribs	

(continued)

Table 10.5 Sternum and Ribs (continued)	
Bone or Bone Marking	**Description**
True ribs	
False ribs	
Floating ribs	

Activity Questions

1. Color the sternum green on the picture below.

2. Color the true ribs blue on the picture below.

3. Color the false ribs red on the picture below.

4. Color the floating ribs yellow on the picture below.

5. Label the following regions of the sternum:
- Manubrium
- Body
- Xiphoid procces

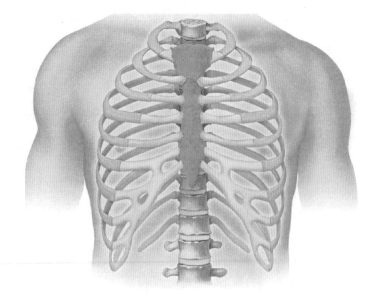

On the images below, fill in the blanks with the bone or bone marking. The parentheses indicate whether you should name the bone or bone marking.

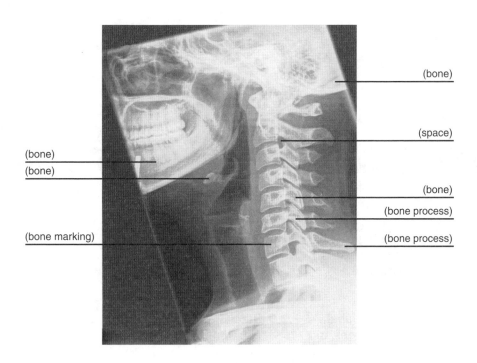

(bone)

(space)

(bone)

(bone)

(bone)

(bone process)

(bone marking)

(bone process)

11

Appendicular Skeleton

Textbook Correlation: Chapter 6—Bones and Joints

Details

Activities	Activity Objectives	Required Materials	Estimated Time
11-1: Bones of the Pectoral Girdle and Upper Appendage	Identify the bones and bone markings of the pectoral girdle and upper appendage.	● Articulated skeleton ● Clavicle ● Scapula ● Humerus ● Ulna ● Radius ● Articulated hand	40 min
11-2: Bone Mapping Part 1	Draw and label various bones and bone markings in the pectoral girdle and upper appendage.	● Butcher paper (very long) ● Pencils ● Markers	40 min
11-3: Bones of the Pelvic Girdle and Lower Appendage	Identify the bones and bone markings of the pelvic girdle and lower appendage.	● Articulated skeleton ● Articulated bony pelvis ● Coxal bones ● Femur ● Patella ● Tibia ● Fibula ● Articulated foot	40 min
11-4: Bone Mapping Part 2	Draw and label various bones and bone markings in the pelvic girdle and lower appendage.	● Body tracing from Activity 11-2 ● Pencils ● Markers	25 min
11-5: Male vs. Female Bony Pelvis	Distinguish between the male and female bony pelvis.	● Articulated female bony pelvis ● Articulated male bony pelvis	10–15 min

Overview

Two people were hiking in the mountains when they stumbled upon a human skeleton. They called the police and investigators arrived at the scene. The forensic anthropologist analyzed the bones and determined that the deceased was a male who either had lifted weights or had been a manual laborer. How did the forensic anthropologist come to these conclusions?

In today's laboratory activities, you will explore the appendicular skeleton, which includes the pectoral and pelvic girdles as well as the upper and lower appendages. You will also play the role of a forensic anthropologist and determine the differences between the male and female bony pelvis.

Need to Know

- **Girdle:**
  - Set of bones that connects the appendage to the axial skeleton
  - **Pectoral girdle:**
    - **Scapula:** commonly known as the shoulder blade; articulates with the humerus (arm bone) and the clavicle
    - **Clavicle:** commonly known as the collarbone; articulates with the sternum (an axial bone)
  - **Pelvic girdle:**
    - Consists of two **coxal** bones that articulate with the sacrum (an axial bone).
    - Each coxal bone is composed of three regions (bones that fuse during childhood): **ilium:** broadest, most superior region; **pubis:** small, inferior, anterior region; **ischium:** small, inferior, posterior region.

- **Bones of the upper appendage:**
  - **Humerus:** long bone found in the arm; its knobby head articulates with the scapula, forming a ball-and-socket synovial joint.
  - **Ulna:** long bone located medially (pinkie-finger side) in the forearm; articulates with the humerus, forming the elbow hinge joint.
  - **Radius:** long bone located laterally (thumb side) in the forearm; articulates with the ulna, forming a pivot joint.
  - **Carpals:** collection of 8 short bones that form the wrist.
  - **Metacarpals:** 5 long bones located in the hand.
  - **Phalanges:** 14 long bones located in the fingers.
    - Four digits (fingers) have three phalanges (proximal, middle, and distal).
    - The thumb has two phalanges (it lacks the middle phalanx).

- **Bones of the lower appendage:**
  - **Femur:** longest bone of the body, located in the thigh; its knobby head articulates with the coxal bones, forming a ball-and-socket joint.
  - **Patella:** a round, short bone that forms the kneecap.
  - **Tibia:** a thick, long bone located medially in the leg; it articulates with the femur, forming the knee hinge joint.
  - **Fibula:** a thin, lateral, non–weight-bearing bone located in the leg.
  - **Tarsals:** a collection of 7 bones that form the ankle.
  - **Metatarsals:** a collection of 8 bones that form the foot.
  - **Phalanges:** a collection of 14 bones found in the toes.
    - Four digits (toes) have three phalanges (proximal, middle, and distal).
    - The great toe has two (it lacks the middle phalanx).

Pre-Lab Activity

Students should complete this activity before completing the lab activities that follow.

1. Define *girdle*.

_____

_____

2. Name the two girdles and name the bones that make up each.

_____

_____

3. Name the articulating bones that connect each girdle to the axial division.

_____

4. Name the collection of "wrist" bones.

_____

_____

5. Name the "kneecap" bone.

_____

6. Most bones in the appendicular skeleton are long bones. Name the three regions of a long bone.

_____

Bones of the Pectoral Girdle and Upper Appendage

Activity Instructions

On the articulated and disarticulated skeletons, identify the bones and bone markings listed in the left-hand column of Table 11.1. As you identify each bone and bone marking, write down a description in the right-hand column. See Figures 6.33 to 6.38 in your textbook (and accomanying narrative).

Table 11.1 Bones of the Pectoral Girdle and Upper Appendage

Bone or Bone Marking	Description
Clavicle	
Scapula	
Scapular spine	
Acromion process	
Coracoid process	
Glenoid cavity (fossa)	
Humerus	
Head	

(continued)

Table 11.1 Bones of the Pectoral Girdle and Upper Appendage (continued)

Bone or Bone Marking	Description
Anatomical neck	
Deltoid tuberosity	
Capitulum	
Trochlea	
Lateral epicondyle (humerus)	
Medial epicondyle (humerus)	
Radial fossa	
Coronoid fossa	
Olecranon fossa	
Ulna	
Olecranon	
Coronoid process	
Trochlear notch	

Table 11.1   Bones of the Pectoral Girdle and Upper Appendage (continued)

Bone or Bone Marking	Description
Radial notch	
Ulnar head	
Ulnar styloid process	
Radius	
Radial head	
Radial tuberosity	
Radial styloid process	
Carpals	
Metacarpals (numbered 1–5, beginning with the thumb)	
Phalanges (*phalanx* is singular)	
Proximal phalanx	
Middle phalanx (not in the thumb)	
Distal phalanx	

Activity Questions

1. Name the posterior fossa on the humerus.

   _____

2. Name the bone marking that forms the pointy elbow. Name the bone that contains the bone marking.

   _____

3. The radial and ulnar styloid processes form the bumps on your wrist. Which one is typically more pronounced (larger)?

   _____

4. Name the bone that is at the very tip of your finger. Be specific.

   _____

5. In the articulated skeleton, does the head of the humerus face medially or laterally? Explain your answer.

   _____

   _____

6. Which arm bone is medial in an articulated skeleton?

   _____

Activity 11-2

Bone Mapping Part 1

This activity consists of tracing the outline of your lab partner's body and then drawing in the anterior view of the bones of the pectoral girdle and upper appendage, as well as various bone markings. The two lab partners then switch places so that the person being traced becomes the tracer. Students may want to draw in the bones and bone markings first in pencil and then draw over the pencil marks with marker.

Activity Instructions

1. Obtain a large piece of butcher paper (the paper should be as long as you are tall).

2. Lie supine (on your back) on the butcher paper with your arms slightly abducted (away from the body) and palms facing the ceiling. Abduct your thigh so that your feet are slightly more than hip width apart.

3. Have another member of the class outline your body with a marker.

4. In pencil, draw and label the bones of the pectoral girdle, arm, forearm, and hand from the anterior view on your outline tracing. Once you are satisfied with your drawing, trace over the pencil with marker. Answer Activity Questions 1, 2, and 3 below.

5. Label the visible fossae on the humerus.

6. Repeat steps 1 to 3 but switch places (the person who outlined is now the person being outlined).

7. Draw and label the bones of the pectoral girdle, arm, and hand from the posterior view on your outline tracing. Answer Activity Question 4 below.

8. Label the olecranon and the ulnar and radial styloid processes.

9. Answer the remaining Activity Questions.

10. Save your mapping exercise for Activity 11-4 later in this lab and also for Activity 18-5 in Laboratory 18.

Activity Questions

1. What bone of the pectoral girdle cannot be seen from the anterior view?

_____

2. Which girdle bone is the most easily palpated and juts out on some individuals?

_____

3. Which forearm bone is on the same side of the arm as the first metacarpal?

_____

4. Should the scapular spine be visible in your drawing? If so, draw it.

_____

5. Which bones generally look the same from both the anterior and posterior views?

_____

6. Which bone is on the same side of the arm as the fifth metacarpal?

_____

Bones of the Pelvic Girdle and Lower Appendage

Activity Instructions

On the articulated and disarticulated skeletons, identify the bones and bone markings listed in the left-hand column of Table 11.2. As you identify the bone and bone marking, write down a description in the right-hand column. See Figures 6.39 to 6.45 in your textbook (and the accompanying narrative).

Table 11.2 Bones of the Pelvic Girdle and Lower Appendage	
Bone or Bone Marking	Description
Coxal bone	
Acetabulum	
Ilium	
Iliac crest	
Posterior superior iliac spine	
Anterior superior iliac spine	
Ischium	
Ischial tuberosity	

Table 11.2 Bones of the Pelvic Girdle and Lower Appendage (continued)

Bone or Bone Marking	Description
Pubic bone	
Pubic symphysis	
Obturator foramen	
Femur	
Femoral head	
Femoral neck	
Femoral shaft (diaphysis)	
Medial condyle (femur)	
Lateral condyle (femur)	
Intercondylar fossa	
Patellar surface	
Tibia	
Medial condyle (tibia)	
Lateral condyle (tibia)	

(continued)

Table 11.2 Bones of the Pelvic Girdle and Lower Appendage (continued)

Bone or Bone Marking	Description
Tibial tuberosity	
Medial malleolus	
Fibula	
Fibular head	
Lateral malleolus	
Patella	
Tarsals	
Talus	
Calcaneous	
Metatarsals (numbered 1–5 beginning with the great toe)	
Phalanges (*phalanx* singular)	
Proximal phalanx	
Middle phalanx (not present in the great toe)	
Distal phalanx	

Activity Questions

1. Name the medial leg bone.

_____

2. What bone are you standing on when you stand on your heels?

_____

3. Does the head of the femur face medially or laterally? Explain your answer.

_____

_____

4. Look at the lateral side of your ankle and then look at the lateral side of the ankle on a skeleton or articulated foot. What bone and bone process form the large bump?

_____

_____

5. Name the bones that form the foot.

_____

Activity 11-4

Bone Mapping Part 2

Activity Instructions

1. Use your body outline tracing from Activity 11-2.

2. Draw and label the pelvic girdle and lower limb bones. If you drew the anterior aspect of the upper appendage, draw the anterior aspect of the pelvic girdle and lower appendage. If you drew the posterior aspect of the upper appendage, draw the posterior aspect of the pelvic girdle and lower appendage.

3. Draw and label the following bone markings:
   - Iliac crest
   - Obturator foramen
   - Acetabulum
   - Tibial tuberosity
   - Intercondylar fossa
   - Medial condyles (all)
   - Lateral condyles (all)
   - Medial malleolus
   - Lateral malleolus

4. Save your bone mapping for Activity 18-5 in Laboratory 18.

Activity Questions

1. Which bone can be seen only from the anterior view?

_____

2. Which of the labeled bone markings can be seen only from the posterior view?

_____

3. Which tibial condyle is on the same side as the head of the femur?

_____

4. Put your hands on your hips and refer to your drawing. What part of the coxal bones are you putting your hands on?

_____

_____

Activity 11-5

Male vs. Female Bony Pelvis

Activity Instructions and Questions

Compare the articulated models of the male and female bony pelvis from different angles.

1. Describe at least three observed structural differences between the male and female bony pelvises.

_____

_____

_____

2. Relate the anatomical differences you noted to differences in function.

_____

_____

_____

Post-Lab Assessment

1. Name the bones in the upper limb from proximal to distal.

   _____

2. Differentiate between the location of the metacarpals and metatarsals.

   _____

3. Name the primary bones that are involved when you type.

   _____

4. Describe how the arm attaches to the axial skeleton, citing specific bone markings.

   _____

   _____

   _____

   _____

   _____

5. Identify the points of articulation between the tibia and the femur.

   _____

6. List the bones of the lower limb from proximal to distal.

   _____

   _____

   _____

7. Name the region of the coxal bones that articulates with the sacrum.

   _____

8. The same regions of the two coxal bones articulate with each other. A small piece of fibrocartilage is located between these two regions. What are these two regions called?

   _____

12

Muscle Tissue and Selected Axial Muscles

Textbook Correlation: Chapter 7—Muscles

Details

Activities	Activity Objectives	Required Materials	Estimated Time
12-1: Muscle Tissue Histology	Differentiate between the three types of muscle tissue; identify various features of the three types of muscle tissue.	• Microscope • Skeletal muscle slide • Cardiac muscle slide • Smooth muscle slide	15 min
12-2: Skeletal Muscle Cell Anatomy	Identify the parts of a muscle cell (fiber).	• Skeletal muscle cell model	15 min
12-3: Neuromuscular Junction Histology	Identify the structures involved in the neuromuscular junction.	• Microscope • Motor end-plate slide	10 min
12-4: Facial Muscles	Identify the muscles of the face; name the origin, insertion, and actions of the muscles of the face.	• Muscular head model • Articulated skeleton with origins and insertions (optional)	25 min

Details (Continued)

Activities	Activity Objectives	Required Materials	Estimated Time
12-5: Muscles Moving the Jaw and Head	Identify the muscles of the jaw and head; name the origin, insertion, and actions of the muscles of the jaw and head.	● Muscular head model ● Articulated skeleton with origins and insertions (optional)	10 min
12-6: Facial Muscle Modeling Activity	Categorize the actions of various facial muscles.	● Articulated skull ● Modeling clay (yellow, purple, green, blue, red)	20 min
12-7: Thoracic and Abdominal Muscles	Identify the muscles of the thorax and abdomen; name the origin, insertion, and actions of the thoracic and abdominal muscles.	● Muscular torso model or muscular whole-body model ● Articulated skeleton with origins and insertions (optional)	25 min
12-8: Muscles of the Perineum	Identify the muscles of the perineum; name the origin, insertion, and actions of the muscles of the perineum.	● Pelvic models (male and female) ● Muscular torso ● Articulated skeleton with origins and insertions (optional)	20 min

Overview

Two students, Deneshia and Liz, were taking a break from studying for their anatomy and physiology exam by working out together on the treadmills at the campus fitness center. "Do you remember whether the muscle in the heart is the same as the muscles that we use to move?" Deneshia asked. "Hmmm . . ." Liz paused. "I think we learned that there are three different types of muscle. Let's see, skeletal for moving the bones, cardiac for the heart. . . . Gosh, I can't remember the third!" Deneshia sighed. "Guess as soon as we finish our workout, we need to get some food and get back to the study hall!"

Can you identify the third type of muscle tissue that Deneshia and Liz couldn't remember? Today's lab focuses on learning about the three types of muscle tissue, the anatomy of a skeletal muscle fiber (cell), and the location and actions of the axial muscles.

Need to Know

There are three types of muscle tissue. Study the table below for details about each.

Characteristic	Skeletal Muscle	Cardiac Muscle	Smooth Muscle
Location	Attached to bones (or the fascia underlying facial skin).	Heart wall.	Surrounds hollow organs (such as blood vessels, stomach, urethra, etc.).
Cell shape	Fiber-shaped (cells are also called **fibers**).	Cylindrical in shape, with branches.	Long and spindle-shaped.
Functional characteristic	Voluntary (can be consciously controlled).	Involuntary (cannot be consciously controlled).	Involuntary (cannot be consciously controlled).
Number of nuclei per cell	Many.	One to two.	One.
Presence of striations (alternating light and dark patterns seen micro-scopically)	Yes.	Yes.	No (hence the name *smooth*).
Other specific characteristics	Each skeletal muscle cell runs the length of the muscle.	**Intercalated discs** are gap junctions between two cardiac cells. They allow for the quick transmission of ions from one cell to another. They appear microscopically as vertical lines between the cells and stain slightly darker than the cell.	Smooth muscle tissue is frequently arranged in two sheets, the circular layer and the longitudinal layer.

● As discussed in Chapter 3, cells have unique structures based on their location and function. Skeletal muscle cells produce force because of the presence of myofilaments, which contain contractile proteins.
  ● **Actin:** found in thin myofilament (along with troponin and tropomyosin)
  ● **Myosin:** found in thick myofilaments
  ● **Z-disc:** located at the ends of the thin filaments
  ● **Sarcomere:** region between two adjacent Z-discs
  ● The names of some cell structures differ:
    ○ **Sarcolemma:** the cell membrane
    ○ **Sarcoplasm:** the cytoplasm
    ○ **Sarcoplasmic reticulum:** the smooth endoplasmic reticulum

- **Somatic motor neuron:**
  - Voluntary neuron that stimulates (excites) skeletal muscle
  - **Axon:** long extension of the nerve cell
    - Extends from the brain or spinal cord to the muscle
    - **Synaptic bulb:** bulb-shaped termination of the axon
  - **Synaptic cleft:** space between the muscle cell and the axon terminal
  - **Motor end plate:** excitable membrane of the skeletal muscle cell
- Skeletal muscle usually attaches to two bones:
  - **Origin:** less movable bone
  - **Insertion:** more movable bone

- **Facial expression muscles:**
  - Responsible for smiling, frowning, grinning, etc.
  - Also responsible for chewing and moving the jaw around.

- **Thoracic cavity muscles:**
  - Essential for respiration (breathing), which involves two phases: inspiration (breathing in) and expiration (breathing out).

- **Abdominal muscles:**
  - Form your core.
  - Incredibly important for virtually any voluntary movement.
  - Weak abdominals typically lead to chronic back pain.

- **Perineal muscles:**
  - Located in the genital region.
  - Regulate a wide variety of functions, such as defecation and erection.

Pre-Lab Activity

Students should complete this activity before completing the lab activities that follow.

1. Name one unique feature of cardiac muscle cells.

   _____

2. What is the cell membrane of skeletal muscle cells called?

   _____

3. Name the only type of muscle tissue that is innervated by a somatic motor neuron.

   _____

4. Name the two contractile proteins found in skeletal muscle.

   _____

5. Which type of muscle cell is long and spindle-shaped?

   _____

6. What is the name for the location of muscle attachment on the more movable bone?

   _____

Muscle Tissue Histology

Activity Instructions

1. Observe skeletal muscle under the microscope (low and high power) and identify the structures listed below. Draw, label, and describe your findings.
   - Skeletal muscle cell (fiber)
   - Striations
   - Nuclei

TM _____

Slide name _____

Description _____

_____

_____

_____

_____

TM _____

Slide name _____

Description _____

_____

_____

_____

_____

2. Observe cardiac muscle under the microscope (low and high power) and identify the structures listed below. Draw, label, and describe your findings.
   ● Cardiac muscle cell
   ● Striations
   ● Intercalated disc
   ● Nuclei

TM _____

Slide name _____

Description _____

_____

_____

_____

_____

TM _____

Slide name _____

Description _____

_____

_____

_____

_____

3. Observe smooth muscle under the microscope (low and high power) and identify the structures listed below. Draw, label, and describe your findings.
- Smooth muscle cell
- Nucleus

TM _____

Slide name _____

Description _____

_____

_____

_____

TM _____

Slide name _____

Description _____

_____

_____

_____

_____

Activity Questions

1. Name the tissue that does not have striations.

_____

2. Name the tissue that has branched cells.

_____

3. Compare the number of nuclei located in the cells of each type of muscle tissue.

_____

_____

_____

4. Both cardiac muscle and skeletal muscle is striated. What is different about the appearance of these two types of muscle tissue?

_____

_____

_____

_____

5. **Critical Thinking:** Cardiac muscle cells are self-stimulating, which means that they do not need a neuron to stimulate contraction. Cardiac muscle also contracts in a synchronous, coordinated fashion because of ion movement from cell to cell through the intercalated discs. Which type of cell junction is found in the intercalated discs?

_____

_____

_____

Activity 12-2

Skeletal Muscle Cell Anatomy

Activity Instructions

On the model of the skeletal muscle cell, identify the structures listed in the left-hand column of Table 12.1. As you identify each structure, write down the corresponding number in the right-hand column. Use Figure 7.2 of the textbook for reference.

Table 12.1 Skeletal Muscles

Name of Structure	Number on Model
Endomysium	
Sarcolemma	
Motor end plate	
Sarcoplasm	
Myofilaments	
Thin filaments (actin)	
Thick filaments (myosin)	
Z-discs	
Sarcomere	
Somatic motor neuron	
Synaptic bulb	

Activity Questions

1. Name the part of the sarcolemma that contains acetylcholine receptors. Hint: It is the part that is separated from the axon terminal by the synaptic cleft.

2. Look at the model of the skeletal muscle fiber. The arrangement of two structures leads to the striations (light and dark banding pattern). Name the two structures.

3. Look at the model of the skeletal muscle fiber. What do you think happens to the length of the sarcomere during contraction?

4. Name the chemical found in the synaptic bulb.

_____

5. Describe the difference between the motor end plate and the sarcolemma.

_____

_____

_____

Activity 12-3

Neuromuscular Junction Histology

Activity Instructions

1. Look at the slide of the motor end plate under the microscope at low and high power. Identify the structures listed below. Draw, label, and describe your findings.
- Skeletal muscle cell
- Motor unit
  - Axon
  - Synaptic bulb

TM _____

Slide name _____

Description _____

_____

_____

_____

_____

TM _____

Slide name _____

Description _____

_____

_____

_____

_____

Activity Questions

1. How many motor neurons innervate one muscle cell?

_____

2. What happens to the axon when it gets close to the muscle cell?

_____

3. Does a voluntary or involuntary motor neuron innervate the skeletal muscle cell?

_____

Facial Muscles

Activity Instructions

On the muscular head model, identify the muscles listed in the left-hand column of Table 12.2. As you identify each muscle, write down the corresponding number in the second column. Also fill in the origin and insertion and muscle action in the other two columns. If you have a hard time finding a particular muscle, use an articulated skeleton with origins and insertions marked on it. If you can locate the origin and insertion on the marked skeleton, it will make it much easier to find the muscle on the model. Refer to Plate 7.1 of the textbook if needed.

Table 12.2 Facial Muscles			
Muscle Name	Number on Model	Origin and Insertion	Muscle Action
Occipitofrontalis			
Frontal belly			
Occipital belly			
Orbicularis oculi			
Nasalis			
Orbicularis oris			
Zygomaticus			
Depressor labii inferioris			
Mentalis			
Depressor anguli oris			
Risorius			
Platysma			

Activity Questions

1. Name one muscle responsible for smiling.

_____

2. Name the muscle that keeps your eyes closed when you are sleeping.

_____

3. Name one muscle that is used when eating.

_____

4. Deeply inhale through your nose. Which facial muscle was activated?

_____

5. Name two muscles responsible for an unhappy face.

_____

Activity 12-5

Muscles Moving the Jaw and Head

Activity Instructions

On the muscular head and torso model, identify the muscles listed in the left-hand column of Table 12.3. As you identify each muscle, write down the corresponding number in the second column. Also fill in the origin and insertion and muscle action in the other two columns. If you have a hard time finding a particular muscle, use an articulated skeleton with origins and insertions marked on it. If you can locate the origin and insertion on the marked skeleton, it will make it much easier to find the muscle on the model. Refer to Plate 7.2 of the textbook if needed.

Table 12.3 Jaw and Head Movement Muscles			
Muscle Name	**Number on Model**	**Origin and Insertion**	**Muscle Action**
Masseter			
Temporalis			
Sternocleidomastoid			
Trapezius			
Erector spinae			
Pterygoids (not described in the textbook)			

Activity Questions

1. Name the muscle that originates from the zygomatic process of the temporal bone and inserts on the mandible.

   _____

2. Name three muscles that move the jaw.

   _____

3. Thrust your jaw forward (anteriorly). Which muscle made that movement?

   _____

4. Name the muscle that originates from the sternum and clavicle and inserts on the mastoid process of the temporal bone.

   _____

Facial Muscle Modeling Activity

This activity will use modeling clay to reinforce the location of the facial and jaw muscles and demonstrate their action.

Activity Instructions

1. Obtain an articulated skull and modeling clay.

2. Get some yellow modeling clay and wrap it around the right eye orbit.

3. Use a piece of purple modeling clay and place it over the zygomatic bone to the corner of the mouth.

4. Wrap a piece of green modeling clay around the mouth (surrounding where the lips would be located).

5. Obtain a piece of blue modeling clay and place it from the corner of mouth (green clay) to the mandible (slightly lateral from the chin).

6. Use a piece of red modeling clay and place it from the zygomatic process of the temporal bone into the mandible.

Activity Questions

1. What muscle does the yellow modeling clay represent? Based on the location, what do you think is the action of this muscle?

   _____

2. What muscle does the purple clay represent? What do you think is the action of this muscle?

   _____

3. Name the muscle represented by the green clay. What is the action of this muscle?

   _____

4. Name the muscle represented by the blue clay. What is the action of this muscle?

   _____

5. What muscle is the red clay representing? What is the action of this muscle?

   _____

Thoracic and Abdominal Muscles

Activity Instructions

On the muscular torso model, identify the muscles listed in the left-hand column of Table 12.4. As you identify each muscle, write down the corresponding number in the second column. Also fill in the origin and insertion and muscle action in the other two columns. If you have a hard time finding a particular muscle, use an articulated skeleton with origins and insertions marked on it. If you can locate the origin and insertion on the marked skeleton, it will make it much easier to find the muscle on the model. Refer to Plate 7.3 of the textbook if needed.

Table 12.4 Thoracic and Abdominal Muscles			
Muscle Name	**Number on Model**	**Origin and Insertion**	**Muscle Action**
Rectus abdominis			
External oblique			
Internal oblique			
Transverse abdominis			

Erector spinae
 	
  Spinalis
 	
  Longissimus
 	
  Iliocostalis			

Diaphragm			
External intercostals			
Internal intercostals			

Activity Questions

1. Take a deep breath without moving your rib cage. Name two muscles responsible for increasing the size of the thoracic cavity.

_____

_____

2. Suck in your abdominal muscles. Which muscles contracted?

_____

_____

3. Name the muscles that are located between the ribs.

_____

4. Name all of the muscles that insert on the xiphoid process of the sternum.

_____

_____

Activity 12-8

Muscles of the Perineum

Activity Instructions

On the muscular torso model, identify the muscles listed in the left-hand column of Table 12.5. As you identify each muscle, write down the corresponding number in the second column. Also fill in the origin and insertion and muscle action in the other two columns. If you have a hard time finding a particular muscle, use an articulated skeleton with origins and insertions marked on it. If you can locate the origin and insertion on the marked skeleton, it will make it much easier to find the muscle on the model. Refer to Plate 7.4 of the textbook if needed.

Table 12.5   Muscles of the Perineum

Muscle Name	Number on Model	Origin and Insertion	Muscle Action
Transverse perineus			
Levator ani			
External anal sphincter			
Ischiocavernosus			
Bulbospongiosus			
Coccygeus			

Activity Questions

1. Name two muscles responsible for erection.

   _____

   _____

2. Name three muscles involved in defecation.

   _____

   _____

3. Name two muscles that originate on the ischial tuberosity.

   _____

   _____

Post-Lab Assessment

1. Differentiate between the sarcomere, sarcolemma, and sarcoplasm.

_____

_____

_____

2. Name the type of muscle tissue that has branched cells.

_____

3. Name the protein bundles found in skeletal muscle cells.

_____

4. Name the most superficial layer of the abdominal muscles.

_____

5. Name two muscles involved in respiration (breathing).

_____

6. Name one muscle that elevates the mandible.

_____

7. Name two muscles that insert on the temporal bone.

_____

8. Label the muscles on the following figures.

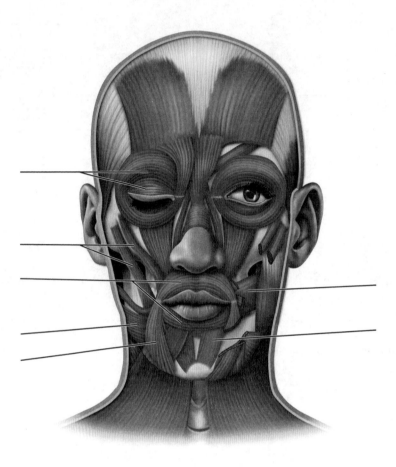

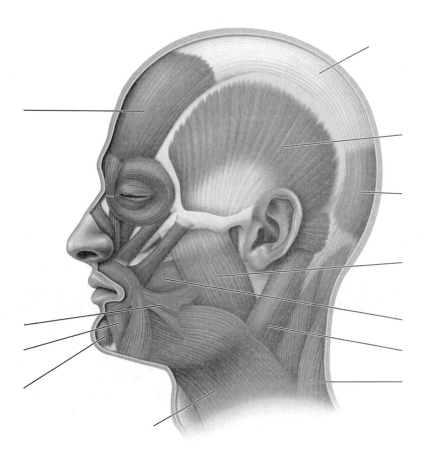

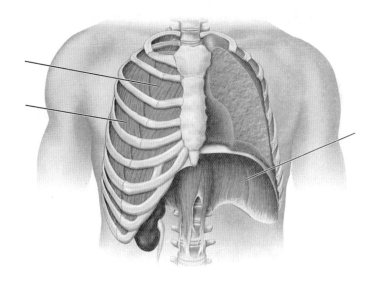

13

Appendicular Muscles

Textbook Correlation: Chapter 7—Muscles

Details

Activities	Activity Objectives	Required Materials	Estimated Time
13-1: Muscles Acting to Move and Stabilize the Pectoral Girdle	Identify the muscles that stabilize and move the pectoral girdle; name the origin, insertion, and action of each muscle.	• Muscular head model • Muscular arm model • Muscular torso model (or whole body) • Articulated skeleton with origins and insertions	20 min
13-2: Muscles Acting at the Shoulder Joint	Identify the muscles that act at the shoulder joint; name the origin, insertion, and action of each muscle.	• Muscular head model • Muscular arm model • Muscular torso model (or whole body) • Articulated skeleton with origins and insertions	20 min
13-3: Muscles Acting at the Forearm, Hand, and Fingers	Identify the muscles that act at the forearm, hand and fingers; name the origin, insertion, and action of each muscle.	• Muscular arm model • Articulated skeleton with origin and insertions	40 min
13-4: Muscles Acting at the Thigh and Leg	Identify the muscles that act at the thigh and leg; name the origin, insertion, and action of each muscle.	• Muscular leg model • Articulated skeleton with origins and insertions	30 min

Details *(Continued)*

Activities	Activity Objectives	Required Materials	Estimated Time
13-5: Muscles Acting on the Foot and Toes	Identify the muscles that act on the foot and toes; name the origin, insertion, and action for each muscle.	• Muscular leg model • Articulated skeleton with origins and insertions	40 min
13-6: Muscle Movement Activity	Review the location and action of selected appendicular muscles.	• Modeling clay (red, purple, blue, yellow, green) • Articulated skeletons	60 min

Overview

At a party celebrating the end of exam week, Julio spent several hours playing an impromptu game of beach volleyball. The next day, he couldn't move his right shoulder and arm without pain. What structures had he injured—bone, joint capsule, ligaments, tendons, muscles? And what makes the shoulder joint particularly susceptible to injury?

This lab examines the muscles that move the bones of the appendicular skeleton. These muscles accomplish movements at synovial joints, such as flexion, extension, and abduction. It is strongly recommended that you review synovial joints and movements prior to this lab.

Need to Know

- The muscles of the upper limb are categorized as muscles that move the
  - **Scapula:**
    - The glenoid fossa of the scapula articulates with the head of the humerus to form the shoulder joint.
    - Movement of the scapula elevates, depresses, retracts, or protracts the shoulder.
  - **Arm:**
    - Muscles originating on the torso move the humerus in respect to the sternum.
    - The shoulder joint permits flexion, extension, abduction, and adduction.
    - The muscles of the rotator cuff help to stabilize the joint.
  - **Forearm:**
    - Muscles originating on the humerus and/or scapula move the forearm (radius and ulna) in respect to the arm (humerus).
    - The elbow **flexors** are located on the anterior side of the arm and forearm, whereas the **extensors** are located on the posterior side of the arm and forearm.
    - The elbow joint also permits pronation and supination.
  - **Wrist:** The wrist joint between the carpals, radius, and ulna is capable of flexion, extension, abduction, and adduction.

- **Fingers:** Joints between metacarpals and phalanges and between phalanges are capable of flexion and extension (and limited abduction/adduction).
- The muscles of the lower limb are categorized as muscles that move the
  - **Thigh:**
    - ○ The head of the femur articulates with the acetabulum of the coxal bone.
    - ○ Muscles originating on the pelvis and vertebrae flex, extend, abduct, and adduct the femur in relation to the pelvis.
  - **Leg:**
    - ○ Muscles originating on the pelvis or femur move the leg (tibia and fibula) relative to the femur.
    - ○ Flexors are in the anterior compartment, extensors are in the posterior compartment.
  - **Foot:** The ankle joint between the tibia, fibula, and talus can perform dorsiflexion, plantarflexion, inversion, and eversion.
  - **Toes:**
    - ○ The joints between the metatarsals and phalanges and between phalanges are capable of flexion and extension (and limited adduction/abduction).
    - ○ Muscles of the leg and foot control the toe joints.

Pre-Lab Activity

Students should complete this activity before completing the lab activities that follow.

1. Name the bones that form the shoulder joint.

   _____

2. Three of the four rotator cuff muscles are named for their location on the scapula—that is, according to the fossa in which they are located. What are the names of the three fossae on the scapula?

   _____

3. Contract your anterior thigh muscles. Which movement occurs at the knee joint?

   _____

4. Contract your anterior arm muscles. Which movement occurs at the elbow joint?

   _____

   _____

Muscles Acting to Move and Stabilize the Pectoral Girdle

Activity Instructions

Identify the following muscles on the muscular neck, muscular arm, and muscular torso models and complete Table 13.1 (the first muscle is filled in for you). Use an articulated skeleton with origins and insertions marked on it when you have a hard time finding a particular muscle. If you can locate the origin and insertion on the marked skeleton, it will make it much easier to find the muscle on the model. Refer to Plate 7.5 of the textbook if needed.

Table 13.1	Pectoral Girdle Muscles			
Muscle Name	**Origin (O) and Insertion (I)**	**Description**	**Number on Model**	**Muscle Action**
Trapezius	O: occipital bone; C7 and thoracic vertebrael: clavicle; acromion and spine of scapula	Large triangular muscle located superficially on the upper back		Elevates and depresses the scapula; rotates the scapula upward
Levator scapulae				
Pectoralis minor				
Rhomboid major				
Serratus anterior				

Activity Questions

Give the appropriate technical name for the movements involved in each of the following actions and explain which muscles are responsible for each.

1. Shrugging the shoulders (that is, raising them up to your ears and then lowering them again).

_____

_____

2. Improving your posture by pulling your shoulders down and back.

_____

_____

Muscles Acting at the Shoulder Joint

Activity Instructions

Identify the following muscles on the muscular neck, muscular arm, and muscular torso models and complete Table 13.2. If you have a hard time finding a particular muscle, use an articulated skeleton with origins and insertions marked on it. If you can locate the origin and insertion on the marked skeleton, it will make it much easier to find the muscle on the model. Refer to Plate 7.6 of the textbook if needed.

Table 13.2 Muscles That Move the Shoulder Joint				
Muscle Name	**Origin and Insertion**	**Description**	**Number on Model**	**Muscle Action**
Latissimus dorsi				
Pectoralis major				
Supraspinatus				
Infraspinatus				
Teres minor				
Subscapularis				
Deltoid				

Activity Questions

1. Julio is experiencing pain radiating from the shoulder, especially when he is rotating the joint laterally. What did Julio most likely injure? What muscles were involved?

_____

_____

_____

2. All of the muscles that move the shoulder joint insert on the same bone. Name the bone.

_____

3. Name the muscle that "caps" the shoulder.

_____

4. Give the appropriate technical name for the movements involved in each of the following actions. Name the muscle responsible for each movement.

   a. Raising your arms to the side of the body, as if doing a jumping jack or making a snow angel.

   _____

   _____

   b. Raising your arms straight in front of you

   _____

   _____

Activity 13-3

Muscles Acting at the Forearm, Hand, and Fingers

Activity Instructions

Identify the following muscles on the muscular arm model and complete Table 13.3. If you have a hard time finding a particular muscle, use an articulated skeleton with origins and insertions marked on it. If you can locate the origin and insertion on the marked skeleton, it will make it much easier to find the muscle on the model. Refer to Plate 7.7 of the textbook if needed.

Table 13.3   Muscles That Move the Forearm, Hand, and Fingers

Muscle Name	Origin and Insertion	Description	Number on Model	Action
Brachialis				
Brachioradialis				
Biceps brachii				
Triceps brachii				
Extensor carpi radialis				
Pronator teres				
Flexor carpi radialis				
Palmaris longus				
Flexor carpi ulnaris				
Flexor digitorum superficialis				
Extensor digitorum				

Activity Questions

1. Give the appropriate technical name for the movements involved in each of the following actions. Name the muscles responsible for each movement.

   a. Clench your fist and hold up your index finger (as in stating that you are #1). What movement is your index finger performing? Which muscles are used for each movement (clenching fist and holding up finger)?

   _____

   _____

   _____

   _____

b. Move your fingers toward your forearm as if you were forming a cup. What movement are your fingers doing? Your wrist? Which muscles are used for the finger and wrist movements?

_____

_____

_____

_____

c. Abduct and adduct your wrist. Which movement is easier? Which muscles are responsible for the easier action?

_____

_____

_____

_____

2. An interesting fact about the palmaris longus is that the presence of the muscle is a genetic trait; not everyone has one! To see if you have the palmaris longus, touch the pads of your first and fifth fingers together and flex your wrist. If a tendon very visibly pops up, you have a palmaris longus. Do the test with your other hand. The presence of the muscle can even vary between your forearms! One forearm can have it and the other can lack the muscle. Was the muscle present? If so, was it present on both forearms or just one?

_____

_____

3. Approximately 10% to 14% of people do not have the palmaris longus. What is the function of the muscle? Are individuals without the muscle at a great disadvantage?

_____

_____

_____

Muscles Acting at the Thigh and Leg

Activity Instructions

Identify the following muscles on the muscular leg model and complete Table 13.4. If you have a hard time finding a particular muscle, use an articulated skeleton with origins and insertions marked on it. If you can locate the origin and insertion on the marked skeleton, it will make it much easier to find the muscle on the model. Refer to Plate 7.8 of the textbook if needed.

Table 13.4 Muscles That Move the Thigh and Leg				
Muscle Name	**Origin and Insertion**	**Description**	**Number on Model**	**Action**
Iliacus				
Psoas				
Sartorius				
Rectus femoris				
Vastus lateralis				
Vastus medialis				
Vastus intermedius				
Gracilis				
Adductor longus				
Adductor magnus				
Pectineus				
Tensor fasciae latae				
Gluteus medius				
Gluteus maximus				
Biceps femoris				
Semitendinosus				
Semimembranosus				

Activity Questions

Give the appropriate technical term for the movement involved in each of the following actions. Name the muscles responsible for the movement.

1. Moving the thigh posteriorly while in a standing position.

_____

_____

2. Moving the foot laterally while standing (thigh muscles only).

_____

_____

3. Moving the leg toward the buttocks and then back to the ground.

_____

_____

4. Lying down on your right side and kicking your thigh up toward the ceiling.

_____

_____

Activity 13-5

Muscles Acting on the Foot and Toes

Activity Instructions

Identify the following muscles on the muscular leg model and complete Table 13.5. If you have a hard time finding a particular muscle, use an articulated skeleton with origins and insertions marked on it. If you can locate the origin and insertion on the marked skeleton, it will make it much easier to find the muscle on the model. Refer to Plate 7.9 of the textbook if needed.

Table 13.5   Muscles That Move the Foot and Toes

Muscle Name	Origin and Insertion	Description	Number on Model	Action
Tibialis anterior				
Extensor digitorum longus				
Extensor hallucis				
Fibularis longus				
Gastrocnemius				
Soleus				
Tibialis posterior				
Flexor digitorum longus				
Flexor hallucis				

Activity Questions

Give the appropriate technical term for the movement involved in each of the following actions. Name the muscles responsible for each movement.

1. Rocking on the ankle side to side (medially and laterally). Which movement has a greater range of motion?

_____

_____

2. Rocking from your toes to your heels. Which movement has a greater range of motion?

_____

_____

3. Jumping up (ascent only).

_____

_____

Muscle Movement Activity

The origin (muscle attachment to the less movable bone) and the insertion (muscle attachment to the more movable bone) are very helpful in determining the movement of the muscle as well as the joint that the muscle moves. For example, the origin of the biceps femoris is the ischial tuberosity and the linea aspera of the femur. It inserts into the head of the fibula and the lateral condyle of the tibia. This information tells you that this muscle moves the leg in relation to the thigh. Remember, the ischium is on the posterior side of the coxal bone; therefore the biceps femoris is found on the posterior side of the thigh, so it must flex the knee joint. The muscle also must move the hip, since it originates on the hip bone.

This activity will reinforce the muscle movements while you use modeling clay as "muscles." Different colors of modeling clay will be placed on an articulated skeleton, extending from the origin to the insertion, representing selected muscles. After "making" the muscle, you will then determine the action of the muscle by its location. This is a closed-book assignment.

Activity Instructions and Questions

1. Work in groups of two to three students.

2. Obtain five different colors of modeling clay and an articulated skeleton.

3. Use the tables that you filled out in the previous activities to determine the origin and insertion of each muscle listed in the tables below.

4. Using the modeling clay color key in the four muscle-group tables below, place the correct color of modeling clay on both the origin and insertion points of the corresponding muscle on the skeleton.

5. Determine the action of the muscle based on its location.

Muscle Group 1: Lower Limb Posterior Muscles

Muscle (color)*	Action
Biceps femoris (red)	
Semitendinosus (purple)	
Gluteus maximus (blue)	
Gastrocnemius (yellow)	
Gracilis (green)	

*Use the left side of the skeleton.

Muscle Group 2: Lower Limb Anterior Muscles

Muscles (color)*	Action
Iliopsoas (red)	
Vastus lateralis (purple)	
Rectus femoris (blue)	
Sartorius (yellow)	
Tibialis anterior (green)	

*Use the right side of the skeleton.

Muscle Group 3: Upper Limb/Torso Posterior Muscles

Muscle (color)*	Action
Latissimus dorsi (red)	
Trapezius (purple)	
Triceps brachii (blue)	
Deltoid (yellow)	
Flexor carpi ulnaris (green)	

*Use the left side of the skeleton.

Muscle Group 4: Upper Limb/Torso Anterior Muscles

Muscle (color)*	Action
Serratus anterior (red)	
Pectoralis major (purple)	
Brachialis (blue)	
Biceps brachii (yellow)	
Brachioradialis (green)	

*Use the right side of the skeleton.

Post-Lab Assessment

1. Color and label the following muscles on the diagram according to the key below:
   a. Levator scapulae: red
   b. Rhomboid minor: yellow
   c. Serratus anterior: purple
   d. Trapezius: orange

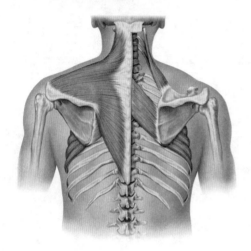

2. Color and label the following muscles on the diagram according to the key below:
   a. Supraspinatus: green
   b. Infraspinatus: orange
   c. Teres major: purple
   d. Teres minor: yellow
   e. Deltoid: blue
   f. Latissimus dorsi: red

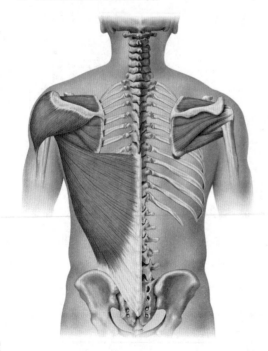

3. Color and label the following muscles on the diagram according to the key below. Note that some muscles can be seen in both views. Color and label the muscle in both views if applicable.
    a. Biceps brachii: blue
    b. Triceps brachii: yellow
    c. Brachioradialis: purple
    d. Palmaris longus: red
    e. Flexor carpi ulnaris: green
    f. Extensor digitorum: orange

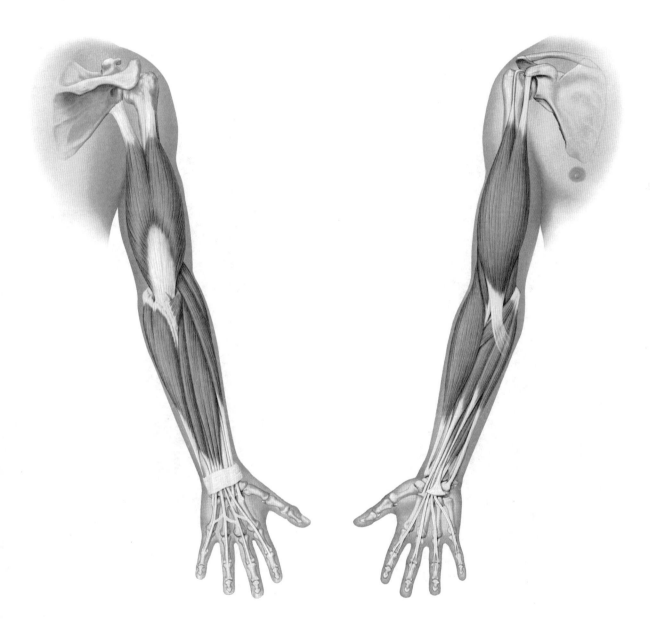

4. Color and label the following muscles on the diagram according to the key below. Note that some muscles can be seen in both views. Color and label the muscle in both views if applicable.

   a. Rectus femoris: red
   b. Biceps femoris: orange
   c. Gracilis: yellow
   d. Sartorius: green
   e. Semitendinosus: blue
   f. Adductor magnus: purple
   g. Vastus medialis: brown

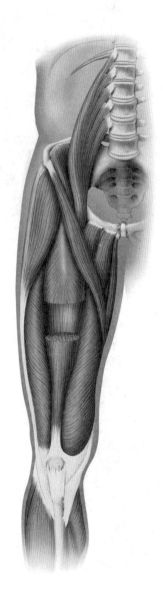
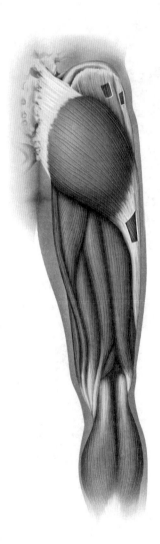

5. Color and label the following muscles on the diagram according to the key below. Note that some muscles can be seen in more than one view.

   a. Fibularis longus: red

   b. Soleus: orange

   c. Flexor digitorum longus: yellow

   d. Tibialis anterior: green

   e. Extensor digitorum: blue

   f. Gastrocnemius: purple

   g. Flexor hallucis: brown

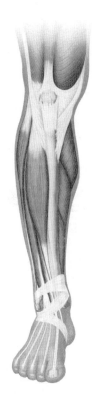
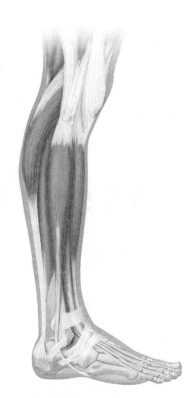
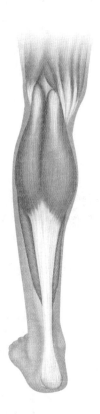
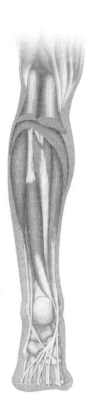

14

Nervous System Histology and Spinal Cord Anatomy

Textbook Correlation: Chapter 4—Communication, and Chapter 8—The Nervous System

Details

Activities	Activity Objectives	Required Materials	Estimated Time
14-1: Neuron Anatomy	Identify the parts of a neuron on both models and microscopic slides	● Neuron model ● Microscope ● Giant multipolar motor neuron slide	20 min
14-2: Build a Neuron	Learn the parts of a neuron by building a model	● Modeling clay in different colors (red, purple, blue, yellow, green)	15 min
14-3: Microscopic Anatomy of a Nerve	Identify the parts of a nerve	● Microscope ● Nerve slide	15 min
14-4: Cross-Sectional Spinal Cord Anatomy	Identify the parts of the spinal cord and related structures located in the PNS*; Name and identify the meninges; Name and identify the parts of the spinal cord microscopically	● Spinal cord cross section (c.s.) model ● Microscope ● Spinal cord (c.s.) slide	15 min

Details *(Continued)*

Activities	Activity Objectives	Required Materials	Estimated Time
14-5: Drawing a Neuron Pathway	Identify the pathways taken by the sensory and motor neurons; Identify the location of cell bodies of sensory and motor neurons	● Colored pencils	15 min
14-6: Longitudinal Anatomy of the Nervous System	Identify the structures of the nervous system in a longitudinal view	● Longitudinal model of the nervous system	15 min

*Peripheral nervous system.

Overview

"Whew, that was close!" Maria thought to herself. She was crossing the street when a car came barreling toward her. She immediately jumped out of the way and was safe from danger. She was excited to attend her next anatomy and physiology class to discuss this instinctive response with her professor. Dr. Avery explained to Maria that her neurons, or excitable cells, allowed her to respond so quickly. Some neurons that stimulate the skeletal muscles participate in reflexes involving the spinal cord—and we jump away from a car before we even have a chance to think about what we're doing. These neuron pathways are particularly adapted to help us escape from danger, and some are so fast that the electrical impulses (signals) can travel at over 100 meters per second! Dr. Avery went on to explain that there are two systems that communicate between parts of the body: the nervous system and the endocrine system. The nervous system is like e-mail: the messages are sent quickly and are electrical. The endocrine system is like a coded message posted on a bulletin board, because hormones are secreted into the bloodstream (where everyone can see them) but only cells that know the code (possess the correct receptor) can respond to the message. Dr. Avery told Maria that they would explore the fascinating world of neurophysiology in lecture and would have an opportunity to observe the anatomy of neurons, nerves, and the spinal cord in the lab.

Like Maria, you will explore in today's lab activities the anatomy of a neuron, a nerve, and the spinal cord as well as structures associated with the spinal cord.

Need to Know

As you most likely remember, there are four general types of tissue: epithelial tissue, connective tissue, muscle tissue, and nervous tissue. We have explored the first three in other lab activities. Today we will focus on nervous tissue.

- Nervous tissue is made up of two types of cells:
  - **Neurons:** conduct electrical impulses through the brain and spinal cord (central nervous system [CNS]) and nerves (peripheral nervous system [PNS]). Neurons have the following parts:
    - ○ **Cell body:** contains the nucleus, mitochondria, lysosomes, Golgi apparatus, and **Nissl bodies,** which are the ribosomes and rough endoplasmic reticulum.
    - ○ **Dendrites:** branching processes that conduct impulses toward the cell body.
    - ○ **Axon:** long process that transmits an impulse away from the cell body.
      - ▪ Some are wrapped by **myelin,** which insulates the axon and increases the speed of impulse conduction.
      - ▪ The **nodes of Ranvier** are axon areas not covered by myelin. The impulse jumps from node to node.
      - ▪ **Axon terminals:** swellings at the end of the axon that store **synaptic vesicles** containing **neurotransmitter.**
  - **Neuroglial cells:** Cells that protect and support neurons

- **Nerves:** bundles of axons in the PNS
  - Contain three membranes
    - ○ Epineurium: surrounds the entire nerve
    - ○ Perineurium: surrounds a small bundle of axons called a fascicle
    - ○ Endoneurium: surrounds each axon (or surrounds the myelin if the axon is in white matter)
  - Organized into networks called **plexuses**
    - ○ **Cervical plexus:** originates from the cervical region and extends to the skin and muscle of the posterior head, neck, and shoulders. It also innervates the diaphragm (through the phrenic nerve).
    - ○ **Brachial plexus:** bundle of nerves that branch and innervate the shoulder and arm.
    - ○ **Lumbar plexus:** bundle of nerves extending from the lumbar region of the spinal cord, innervating a portion of the lower limb, abdominal wall, and external genitalia.
    - ○ **Sacral plexus:** nerves that extend from the sacral region innervating most of the lower limb, buttocks, and perineum.
  - **Intercostal nerves:** take the place of a thoracic plexus; the nerves run through the intercostal muscles.

- **Spinal cord:** transmits impulses to and from the brain and is a reflex center.
  - Terminates as the **cauda equina** (horse's tail)
  - Covered by protective membranes called **meninges**
    - ○ **Dura mater:** most superficial meningeal layer
    - ○ **Arachnoid:** middle meningeal layer
    - ○ **Pia mater:** thin membrane that is in direct contact with the spinal cord.
  - The following structures are visible in cross section:
    - ○ **Subarachnoid space:** the space deep to the arachnoid in which cerebrospinal fluid (CSF) circulates.
    - ○ **Epidural space:** the space between the dura and the bone that is typically filled with adipose tissue. "Epidurals" are injections inserted into the epidural space in the lower lumbar region.
  - Contains two types of nervous tissue:
    - ○ **Gray matter:** H-shaped tissue in the middle of the spinal cord.
      - ■ **Dorsal horns (2):** contain sensory neurons.
      - ■ **Ventral horns (2):** contain motor neurons.
      - ■ **Central canal:** runs through the gray matter and is lined with ciliated **ependymal cells** (a type of neuroglial cell) that facilitate circulation of CSF.
    - ○ **White matter (tracts):** posterior columns are superficial to the dorsal gray horns; anterior columns are superficial to the ventral gray horns.
      - ■ **Posterior median sulcus:** shallow indentation in the posterior column
      - ■ **Anterior median fissure:** deep indentation in the anterior column

- **PNS structures related to the spinal cord**
  - **Dorsal root:** contains axons of sensory neurons entering the dorsal horn
    - ○ **Dorsal root ganglion:** collection of cell bodies of sensory neurons
  - **Ventral root:** contains axons of motor neurons exiting from the ventral horn
    - ○ There is no ventral root ganglion, since the cell bodies of motor neurons are located in the ventral horn.
  - **Spinal nerves:** contain both sensory and motor neurons
    - ○ Formed by the merger of the dorsal and ventral roots
    - ○ Divide into three branches:
      - ■ Dorsal branch: innervates skin and muscles of the back
      - ■ Ventral branch: innervates skin and muscles of the anterior body
      - ■ Communicating branches (only certain nerves): carry sympathetic neurons only

Pre-Lab Activity

Students should complete this activity using their textbook for reference before completing the lab activities that follow.

1. Draw a picture of a neuron and label the parts.

2. Color the figure of a cross section of a nerve according to the following color scheme:
- Epineurium: orange
- Perineurium: blue
- Fascicles: yellow
- Myelin: white
- Axon: red

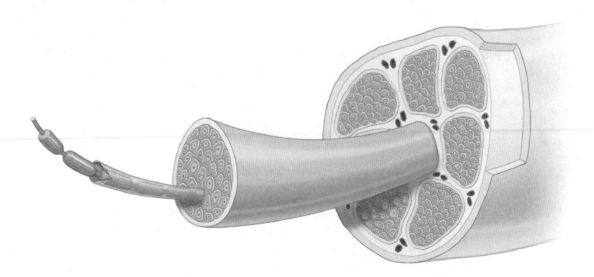

3. Describe the difference between a neuron and a nerve.

_____

_____

_____

4. Color the figure of a cross section of the spinal cord according to the following color scheme:
- Dorsal branch: red
- Ventral branch: orange
- Spinal nerve: yellow
- Dorsal root ganglion: green
- Dorsal root: blue
- Dorsal horns: purple
- Ventral horns: pink
- Ventral root: brown
- Label the white columns

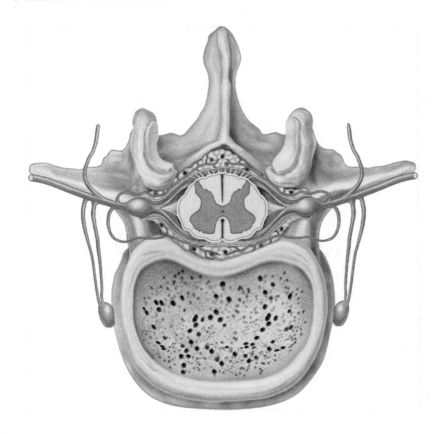

5. Color the following structures on the diagram according to the colors listed below.

- Spinal cord: red
- Cauda equina: pink
- Cervical plexus: green
- Brachial plexus: purple
- Intercostal nerves: orange
- Lumbar plexus: blue
- Sacral plexus: yellow

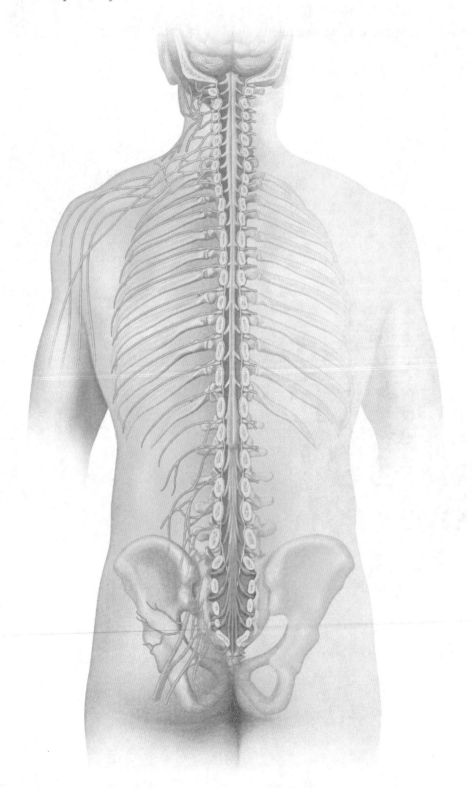

Neuron Anatomy

Activity Instructions

1. Identify the following structures on the neuron model. Refer to Figure 4.7 in Chapter 4 of the text. Fill in Table 14.1.

Table 14.1 Neuron Model Structures	
Name of Structure	**Corresponding Number on Model**
Dendrites	
Cell body	
Nucleus	
Mitochondria	
Axon	
Schwann cell	
Myelin	
Node of Ranvier	
Axon terminal	

2. Obtain a giant multipolar motor neuron slide and a microscope. View the slide under high power. Identify the structures listed below. Draw, label, and describe what you are viewing.
   - Cell body
   - Processes (can't really distinguish between an axon and the dendrites)
   - Nuclei of neuroglial cells (small dots seen throughout the field of view)

TM _____

Slide name _____

Description _____

_____

_____

_____

_____

Activity Questions

1. Which structure carries information toward the cell body?

   _____

2. Which structure conducts an impulse away from the cell body?

   _____

3. **Critical Thinking:** Neurons are amitotic (incapable of undergoing mitosis) because they lack one cell organelle necessary for replication. Think back to the mitosis lab. What cell organelle are they lacking?

   _____

Build a Neuron

In this activity, you will build a neuron out of modeling clay. Different colors of clay will represent different structures of the neuron.

Activity Instructions

1. Obtain five different colors of modeling clay (red, purple, blue, white, and green).

2. Use the purple modeling clay and roll it into a ball. That is the cell body.

3. Get several small pieces of red modeling clay and roll each out so that it is short and skinny (like spikes).

4. Attach the red spikes to the cell body.

5. Use a piece of the blue modeling clay and roll it out into a long, skinny, snake-like structure. Attach it to the cell body, in an area that does not contain the red spikes.

6. Answer Activity Questions 1 and 2 below.

7. Get some white modeling clay and wrap it around the blue structure, ensuring that there are some spaces or parts of exposed blue. This white structure represents the myelin sheath.

8. Answer Activity Questions 3 and 4 below.

9. Obtain some green modeling clay. Wrap the green modeling clay around the distal portion of the myelin. This represents a thin fibrous membrane. Answer the remaining Activity Questions.

Activity Questions

1. What structures do the red spikes represent?

    _____

2. What structure does the long, skinny, snake-like structure represent?

    _____

3. If this neuron were in the PNS, what cell would form the myelin?

    _____

4. What are the exposed blue areas called?

    _____

5. What is the name of the membrane represented by the green clay?

_____

6. If the whole class put their blue structures together, what would that bundle be called?

_____

7. What would the bundle be called if we made it smaller and wrapped it in perineurium?

_____

Activity 14-3

Microscopic Anatomy of a Nerve

This activity allows you to view a nerve microscopically and identify the parts of a nerve. Refer to Figure 8.5 of the textbook or your coloring exercise in the pre-lab activity.

Activity Instructions

1. Obtain a nerve slide and view it under both low- and high-power magnifications. Identify the structures listed below. Draw, label, and describe your findings.
- Epineurium
- Nerve
- Perineurium
- Fascicle
- Endoneurium
- Myelin
- Axon

TM _____

Slide name _____

Description _____

_____

_____

_____

_____

_____

TM _____

Slide name _____

Description _____

_____

_____

_____

_____

TM _____

Slide name _____

Description _____

_____

_____

_____

_____

Activity Questions

1. How many fascicles do you observe making up one nerve?

_____

2. What is the name of the fibrous membrane surrounding the fascicle?

_____

3. What is the smallest unit of a nerve?

_____

4. Would this slide be a sample from the PNS or CNS? Explain your answer.

_____

_____

_____

Activity 14-4

Cross-Sectional Spinal Cord Anatomy

Activity Instructions

1. Identify the structures listed in Table 14.2 on the cross-sectional model of the spinal cord and related structures, using Figure 8.16 of the textbook as a guide. Indicate whether the structure is part of the CNS or PNS.

Table 14.2 Cross-Sectional Spinal Cord Anatomy and Related Structures

Name of Structure	Nervous System Division	Corresponding Number on Model
Anterior median fissure		
Central canal		
Communicating branch		
Dorsal horns		
Dorsal branch		
Dorsal root		
Dorsal root ganglion		
Dura mater		
Epidural space filled with adipose tissue		
Pia mater		
Posterior median sulcus		
Spinal nerve		
Subarachnoid space		
Sympathetic chain ganglion		
Ventral branch		
Ventral horns		
Ventral root		
White columns (anterior and posterior)		

2. Obtain a spinal cord slide and view it under scanning, low-, and high-power magnifications. Identify the structures listed below. Draw, label, and describe your findings.
   - Dorsal horns
   - Ventral horns
   - White columns (anterior and posterior)
   - Central canal
     - Ependymal cells

TM _____

Slide name _____

Description _____

_____

_____

_____

_____

TM _____

Slide name _____

Description _____

_____

_____

_____

_____

TM _____

Slide name _____

Description _____

_____

_____

_____

_____

Activity Questions

1. Is the ventral root ganglion part of the PNS or the CNS? Explain your answer.

_____

_____

_____

_____

2. Name the most superficial meningeal membrane.

_____

3. The central canal circulates a fluid around the spinal cord and brain. Name the fluid that is circulated throughout the central canal.

_____

Activity 14-5

Drawing a Neuron Pathway

Activity Instructions

Follow the instructions below by drawing lines on the accompanying illustration.

1. Using a purple pencil, draw a line on the right side of the picture, going through the dorsal branch, spinal nerve, dorsal root ganglion, dorsal root, dorsal horn, and superior portion of the ventral horn. Draw an inverted "V" to represent a synapse.

2. Answer Activity Questions 1 and 2.

3. Use an orange colored pencil to draw a line on the right side of the picture, going from the ventral horn, through the ventral root, spinal nerve, and then through the dorsal branch.

4. Answer Activity Questions 3 to 5.

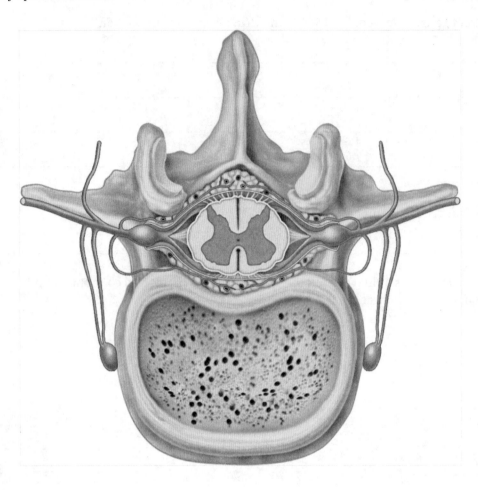

Activity Questions

1. What type of information does the purple neuron convey?

_____

2. Where should you put the cell body of the purple neuron? Write your answer here and add it to your drawing.

_____

3. What type of information does the orange neuron convey?

_____

4. Where should you draw the cell body of the orange neuron? Write your answer here and add it to your drawing.

_____

5. Give a specific example of an effector organ that the motor neuron would stimulate (remember, it is traveling through the dorsal branch).

_____

6. According to your drawing, what structure(s) do both sensory and motor neurons pass through?

_____

Activity 14-6

Longitudinal Anatomy of the Nervous System

Activity Instructions

Identify the structures listed in Table 14.3 on the longitudinal model of the nervous system, using Figure 8.17 of the textbook as a guide. Fill in the right-hand column of the table.

Table 14.3 Longitudinal Nervous System Anatomy

Name of Structure	Correlating Number on Model
Spinal cord	
Anterior median fissure	
Dorsal root ganglion	
Sympathetic chain ganglion	
Communicating branches	
Cervical plexus	
Phrenic nerve	
Brachial plexus	
Lumbar plexus	
Sacral plexus	
Sciatic nerve	
Intercostal nerves	

Activity Questions

1. What are the long extensions of the spinal nerves at the end of the spinal cord called?

_____

2. Name one general area of the body that each plexus innervates:

   a. Cervical plexus:_____

   b. Brachial plexus: _____

   c. Lumbar plexus: _____

   d. Sacral plexus: _____

Post-Lab Assessment

1. Name the cells that line the central canal.

_____

2. Name the cells that wrap around the axon. Name the structure they form. Name the membrane that is superficial to the axon.

_____

3. Name the meningeal layers from deep to superficial.

_____

4. Which is the sensory area of the spinal cord—dorsal or ventral? Explain your answer.

_____

_____

_____

5. **Critical Thinking:** A specific disease affects the meninges and is caused by either bacteria or viruses. The viral form of this disease is typically curable, but the bacterial form is typically deadly. Signs typically include a very high fever and excruciating pain in the neck and head. Inflammation is a key factor. Both forms are highly contagious. The disease is confirmed via a spinal tap.

   a. Based on the information above, what disease do you think affects the meninges in this way? (Hint: the suffix –*itis* indicates inflammation).

   _____

   b. The disease is detected via a spinal tap whereby some fluid is withdrawn by a very large needle. What fluid do you think is sampled? Where on the spinal cord do you think the spinal tap is performed? Explain your answer. (Hint: it is performed in a location where the least amount of damage will occur.)

   _____

   _____

   _____

15

Brain and Cranial Nerve Anatomy; Reflexes

Textbook Correlation: Chapter 8—The Nervous System

Details

Activities	Activity Objectives	Required Materials	Estimated Time
15-1: Brain Anatomy	Identify the regions and structures of the brain.	• Brain model	25 min
15-2: Meninges	Identify the meningeal membranes and describe the folds in the dura mater.	• Brain model • Paper towels	10 min
15-3: Ventricles	Identify the components of the ventricular system; Trace the flow of CSF.*	• Ventricle model and/or • Brain model	10 min
15-4: Identification of Cranial Nerves	Identify, by both number and name, the 12 cranial nerves.	• Brain model	15 min
15-5: Sheep Brain Dissection	Identify the regions and structures of the sheep brain, including the folds of the dura mater (if applicable).	• Sheep brain (1 per group of 4 students)	20–30 min (depending on whether the dura mater is present)

Details *(Continued)*

Activities	Activity Objectives	Required Materials	Estimated Time
15-6: Assessment of Cranial Nerve Function	Describe the function of cranial nerves.	● Several fragrant items (such as coffee grounds, lemon, cinnamon, etc.) ● Blindfold ● Snellen eye examination chart ● Flashlight ● Cotton balls ● Pen cap	60 min
15-7: Reflex Activity	Apply the principles of reflexes; explain how factors affect the strength of reflexes as well as reaction time.	● Percussion hammer ● Meter stick	15 min

*Cerebrospinal fluid.

Overview

Shanna was driving home from night class when a drunk driver hit her head-on. Shanna had her seat belt on and survived but was unconscious when emergency vehicles arrived on scene. The paramedics strapped her to a C-spine immobilizer to keep her body stable and rushed her to the hospital. Upon admittance to the hospital, an MRI of her brain was ordered. The radiologist used his knowledge of brain anatomy to localize the trauma to two specific brain regions: the *prefrontal cortex* and the *motor cortex*. The neurologist performed a variety of tests, which suggested that Shanna's ability to plan and carry out movements was impaired. However, the head trauma did not damage any cranial nerves.

Today's lab investigates the structure and function of the brain and cranial nerves.

Need to Know

● The **brain** is made up of four regions:
  ● **Cerebrum:** the largest, convoluted region
    ○ Surface features: bumps called *gyri* and grooves called *sulci; fissures* are very deep sulci.
    ○ Divided into left and right cerebral hemispheres by the *longitudinal fissure*.
    ○ Further divided into lobes with the same names as the cranial bones.
    ○ Contains both gray matter (*cortex, nuclei*) and white matter (*tracts*).
  ● **Diencephalon:** small region deep to the cerebrum containing the
    ○ **Thalamus:** almond-shaped structure
    ○ **Hypothalamus:** triangular region anterior and slightly inferior to the thalamus; contains the **mamillary body**
    ○ **Pineal gland:** the knob at the posterior base of the thalamus

- **Brainstem:** resembles the body of a seahorse, composed of the:
  - ○ **Midbrain:** head and neck of seahorse (**superior** and **inferior colliculi:** the two bumps located on the posterior side of the neck of the seahorse)
  - ○ **Pons:** the pudgy portion of the seahorse
  - ○ **Medulla oblongata:** the slender inferior tail of the seahorse
- **Cerebellum:** the ball-shaped structures that project from the inferior and posterior portion of the cerebrum

- **Meninges:** the protective membranes that also cover the spinal cord (see Lab 14). The thick dura mater extends into the large fissures to form folds.
  - **Falx cerebri:** extends down the longitudinal fissure between the two cerebral hemispheres
  - **Tentorium cerebelli:** fold of the dura mater forming a partition between the posterior cerebrum and the cerebellum

- **Ventricular system:** hollow cavities (spaces) in the brain through which CSF circulates
  - **Lateral ventricles:** two spaces shaped like a ram's horn
  - **Third ventricle:** space between the two halves of the diencephalon
  - **Fourth ventricle:** small triangular space between the brainstem and the cerebellum
  - **Cerebral aqueduct:** small, slender tube that connects the third and fourth ventricles
  - **Choroid plexus:** modified blood vessels located in each ventricle that produce and secrete CSF at the same rate at which it is absorbed into venous blood

- **Cranial Nerves:** Twelve cranial nerves project from the brain and cervical spinal cord (see list in Activity 15-4 and Figure 8.14 in your textbook).

- **Reflexes:** rapid, predictable responses to certain stimuli. Listed below are the components of a simple reflex arc.
  - Sensory receptor: structure that detects a stimulus (change in the environment).
  - Sensory (afferent) neuron: transmits sensory information from the sensory receptor to the integration center.
  - Integration center (spinal cord, sometimes brain): interprets the sensory information and sends command to the motor neuron.
  - Motor (efferent) neuron: transmits motor information from the spinal cord to the effector.
  - Effector: structure that is activated to respond to the stimulus. In a somatic reflex, the effector is skeletal muscle; in a visceral reflex, the effector is smooth muscle, cardiac muscle, or a gland.

Pre-Lab Activity

Students should complete this activity before completing the lab activities that follow.

1. Name the fluid that circulates through the ventricular system.

_____

2. True or False: If the statement is false, describe why it is false.

_____"Cranial nerves are part of the central nervous system (CNS)."

_____

_____

_____

3. Color the lobes of the cerebrum according to the key listed below:
  ● Frontal lobe: blue
  ● Parietal lobe: green
  ● Occipital lobe: red
  ● Temporal lobe: yellow
  ● Label the central sulcus (the groove that separates the frontal and parietal lobes).

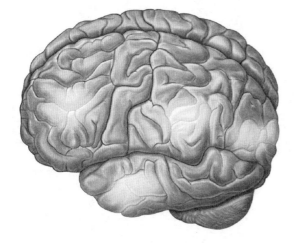

4. On the figure below, draw lines separating the following:
   - Thalamus from hypothalamus
   - Midbrain from pons
   - Pons from medulla oblongata

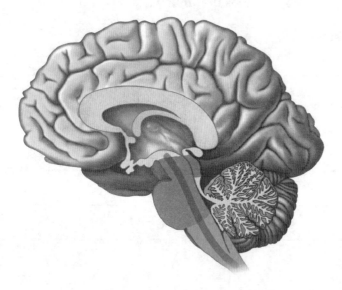

5. On the figure above, label the four regions of the brain and color each region according to the following color scheme:
   - Cerebrum: purple
   - Diencephalon: orange
   - Brainstem: green
   - Cerebellum: red

Brain Anatomy

Activity Instructions

On the brain model, identify the structures listed in the left-hand column of Table 15.1. As you identify each structure, write down the corresponding number in the right-hand column, using textbook Figures 8.8 and 8.13 as guides. Indicate the brain region (cerebrum, diencephalon, brainstem or cerebellum) for each structure.

Table 15.1 Brain Model		
Name of Structure	**Brain Region**	**Corresponding Number on Model**
Cerebral hemispheres (right and left)		
Cerebral cortex		
Cingulate gyrus		
Central sulcus		
Lateral sulcus		
Longitudinal fissure		
Transverse fissure		
Frontal lobe		
Parietal lobe		
Occipital lobe		
Temporal lobe		

(continued)

Table 15.1 Brain Model (continued)		
Name of Structure	Brain Region	Corresponding Number on Model
Insula		
Corpus callosum		
Thalamus		
Hypothalamus		
Mamillary body		
Pineal gland		
Cerebral peduncles		
Superior colliculus		
Inferior colliculus		
Pons		
Medulla		
Cerebellar peduncles		
Cerebellar cortex		
Arbor vitae (white matter)		

Activity Questions

1. Name the structure that separates the frontal and parietal lobes.

   _____

2. Name the structure that allows for communication between the right and left cerebral hemispheres.

   _____

3. Name the structure that is inferior to the pons.

   _____

4. The cerebral cortex is composed of gray matter. Name three parts of a neuron you would expect to see in gray matter.

   _____

5. **Critical Thinking:** Think back to the bones of the skull. How do the sizes of the frontal and parietal lobes compare to those of the frontal and parietal bones? Explain a possible reason for the discrepancy in size.

   _____

   _____

   _____

   _____

   _____

   _____

   _____

Meninges

The meninges consist of three membranes that protect the brain. See textbook Figure 8.6 for more information.

Activity Instructions and Questions

Obtain a brain model and a paper towel.

1. Touch the cerebral cortex. What meningeal layer are you touching?

   _____

2. Which membrane appears "cobwebby"?

   _____

3. Fold your paper towel in half longitudinally. Place the folded part in the longitudinal fissure, letting the two halves of the paper towel drape over the model. What fold of the dura mater is represented by the paper towel in the longitudinal fissure?

   _____

4. Name the vein found in the fold above.

   _____

5. Remove the paper towel from the longitudinal fold and place the folded section between the cerebrum and the cerebellum. What fold of the dura mater is represented now?

   _____

Ventricles

Recall that the ventricles produce and circulate CSF. See textbook Figure 8.7 for more information.

Activity Instructions

On the ventricle or brain model, identify the structures listed in the left-hand column of Table 15.2. As you identify each structure, write down the corresponding number in the right-hand column. Remember that the ventricles are spaces in the brain; the ventricle model represents a cast of the spaces in the brain.

Table 15.2 Ventricles and Related Structures	
Structure	**Corresponding Number on Model**
Choroid plexus	
Lateral ventricles (first and second ventricles)	
Third ventricle	
Cerebral aqueduct	
Fourth ventricle	

Activity Questions

1. Name the neuroglial cells that line the ventricles in order to facilitate the circulation of CSF. Hint: These cells also line the central canal of the spinal cord.

_____

2. Trace the flow of CSF from its production in the choroid plexus of the first ventricle, through the entire ventricular system, to the superior sagittal sinus. Assume that the CSF does not enter the central canal of the spinal cord.

_____

_____

_____

Identification of Cranial Nerves

Activity Instructions

On the brain model, identify the cranial nerves listed in the left-hand column of Table 15.3. As you identify each structure, write down the corresponding number in the right-hand column. Use textbook Figure 8.14 for help.

Table 15.3 Nerves	
Cranial Nerve	**Corresponding Number on Model**
I: Olfactory nerve	
II: Optic nerve	
III: Oculomotor nerve	
IV: Trochlear nerve	
V: Trigeminal nerve	
VI: Abducens nerve	
VII: Facial nerve	
VIII: Vestibulocochlear nerve	
IX: Glossopharyngeal nerve	
X: Vagus nerve	
XI: Accessory nerve	
XII: Hypoglossal nerve	

Activity Questions

1. Work with your classmates to think of a mnemonic using the first letters of the cranial nerves in order. Write it here.

_____

_____

_____

2. Name the cranial nerves that carry sensory information.

_____

_____

_____

3. Name the cranial nerves that primarily carry motor information.

_____

_____

_____

4. Describe the location and anatomical relationship between the abducens, facial, and vestibulocochlear nerves.

_____

_____

_____

Sheep Brain Dissection

Activity Instructions

1. Obtain the necessary dissection supplies (dissecting tray/pan, scalpel, scissors, gloves).

2. Put on the gloves and obtain one sheep brain per each group of four students.

3. Observe the dorsal surface of the brain and identify the following structures:
   - Optic nerve
   - Pituitary gland (hypophysis)

Follow the steps below if your brain has the dura mater intact. Proceed to step 10 if the dura mater has already been removed.

4. Rotate the brain so that you are looking at the ventral surface.

5. Take the scissors and start cutting the dura mater. It is best to begin cutting laterally (either on the right or left side) to the falx cerebri and work your way anteriorly and posteriorly, stopping at the occipital lobe and frontal lobe.

6. Turn the brain dorsally and cut the dura mater around the olfactory bulbs and from the right to left sides of the brain, so that the ventral dura mater is separated from the dorsal dura mater.

7. Once you have made a cut through the ventral surface of the dura mater, carefully peel the falx cerebri out of the longitudinal fissure. If you do this carefully and gently, you will be able to see the superior sagittal sinus.

8. Hold the brain so that the cerebellum is facing you and gently pull the freed ventral dura mater toward you, allowing you to view the tentorium cerebelli.

9. Remove the rest of the dura mater, using the scissors. Don't worry if you remove the optic nerves and the pituitary gland in the process.

10. Identify the following structures:
    - Frontal lobe
    - Parietal lobe
    - Temporal lobe
    - Occipital lobe
    - Cerebellum
    - Pons
    - Medulla oblongata

11. Hold the brain so that the cerebellum is facing you. Very gently, pull the cerebellum back to expose the posterior side of the midbrain and identify the:
    - Superior colliculi
    - Inferior colliculi

12. Place the brain ventrally on the dissecting tray. Take the scalpel and make a midsagittal incision through the longitudinal fissure, cerebellum, and brainstem. When you are done, you should have two equal halves of the brain.

13. Identify the following structures:
    ● Corpus callosum
    ● Lateral ventricle (you will have to poke through a very thin membrane called the septum pellucidum in order to view the space.)
        ● Choroid plexus (visible in a good specimen and cut)
    ● Thalamus
    ● Hypothalamus
    ● Pineal gland
    ● Superior colliculus
    ● Inferior colliculus
    ● Pons
    ● Medulla oblongata
    ● Cerebellum
        ● Arbor vitae

Activity Questions

1. How does the ratio of the size of the pineal gland to the size of the sheep brain compare with that of the human brain models? Based on the function of the pineal gland, what do you think are the ramifications of this difference in size ratio? Hint: The pineal gland secretes melatonin, which induces sleepiness.

_____

_____

_____

_____

2. In the sheep brain, which was larger: the superior colliculi or the inferior colliculi? Based on the function of each, what do you think that means? Hint: The superior colliculus controls the visual startle reflex, whereas the inferior colliculus controls the auditory startle reflex.

_____

_____

_____

_____

Assessment of Cranial Nerve Function

Activity Instructions

The following lab exercise will assess the function of the cranial nerves through a series of tests. Work with a partner, and decide who will be the subject. If time permits, switch roles.

Cranial Nerve I: Olfactory Nerve

1. Put a blindfold over the subject's eyes.

2. Instruct the subject to occlude the right nostril.

3. Place several everyday objects (nonirritating), one at a time, under the subject's open nostril and ask him or her to identify the object. (Examples of items: coffee grounds, vanilla extract, rubbing alcohol, cinnamon, and so on.)

4. Record the subject's responses in Table 15.4.

5. Repeat the test with the left nostril and record the data in Table 15.5.

   ● If the subject can accurately identify each smell using either nostril, cranial nerve I (CN I) is healthy.

Table 15.4 Olfactory Nerve Data: Right Nostril	
Actual Item/Scent	**Subject's Response**

Table 15.5 Olfactory Nerve Data: Left Nostril	
Actual Item/Scent	**Subject's Response**

Cranial Nerve II: Optic Nerve

Visual Acuity

1. Have the subject stand 20 feet away from the Snellen eye examination chart. Instruct him or her to remove glasses (if applicable), close the right eye, and cover it with the right hand. Tell the subject to read as many rows as he or she can, starting with the big letter "E." Record the number of the last line that was identified correctly. Record the number below:

   a. Left eye acuity: 20/_____

2. Repeat the above instructions, but this time the subject is asked to close and cover the left eye.

   a. Right eye acuity: 20/_____

3. Normal vision is 20/20. How do the results in each eye compare with normal vision? How do the eyes compare with each other?

   _____

   _____

Visual Fields

1. Stand approximately 2 feet in front of the subject and instruct him or her to maintain steady eye contact with you. Instruct the subject to tell you which finger is wriggling as soon as it is observed. Spread out your arms 2 feet laterally to the subject's ears, wriggling your fingers and moving your arms closer to the subject until the finger wriggling has been observed. Record your findings below.

   _____

   _____

   _____

2. Repeat the test, but place your arms in the upper temporal quadrant (more superior than ear level). Record your findings below.

_____

_____

_____

_____

3. Repeat the test again, this time placing your arms in the lower temporal quadrant (about chin level). Record your findings below.

_____

_____

_____

_____

● **If the subject can see the fingers peripherally in all locations tested, cranial nerve II (CN II) is healthy.**

Cranial Nerve III: Oculomotor Nerve

1. Instruct the subject to focus on an image several feet away.

2. Turn on a flashlight and flash the light at an angle (not directly) into the subject's **left** eye while observing the response of the **left** eye. Record your observations below.

_____

_____

3. Repeat the above instructions (shine the light at an angle into the **left** eye), but this time observe the response in **right** eye. Record your observations below.

_____

_____

4. Repeat the test again, this time flashing the light into the **right** eye. Observe the response of the **right** eye. Record your observations below.

_____

_____

5. Repeat the exam one more time by flashing the light in the **right** eye, but observe the response in the **left** eye. Record your observations below.

_____

_____

● If both pupils constrict in response to light entering either eye, cranial nerve III (CN III) is healthy.

Cranial Nerves III, IV, VI: Oculomotor Nerve, Trochlear Nerve, and Abducens Nerve

1. Tell the subject to track (follow) your finger while keeping his or her head still.

2. Move your finger in the shape of an "H" while the subject tracks your finger. Observe both of the subject's eyes following your finger. Record your findings below.

_____

_____

_____

3. Again, the subject will track your finger. Test for eye convergence by moving your finger toward the bridge of the subject's nose while observing the movement of both of the subject's eyes. The eyes should come together. Record your findings below:

_____

_____

_____

● If both eyes can track your finger and they converge as the finger moves closer to the bridge of the nose, CN II, IV, and VI are healthy.

Cranial Nerve V: Trigeminal Nerve

Sensory Assessment

1. Lightly swipe a piece of cotton against the subject's right cheek while his or her eyes are closed. Tell the subject to inform you once the cotton is felt. Record if the subject felt the cotton immediately or if it took some time.

_____

2. Repeat the above, this time swiping the cotton on the left check. Record how quickly the subject felt the cotton and if there was any discrepancy from the right side.

_____

_____

_____

3. Tell the subject to close his or her eyes during this series of tests. Obtain a pen cap. There are two sides to the pen cap: the "sharp" side, which has the pointy process, and the "dull" side, or the other end that completely seals the pen. Tap the sharp and dull surfaces against the right side of the subject's forehead (you don't have to alternate the two surfaces; in fact, it is best to randomize the surfaces). After each tap, the subject should state if is the object feels like a sharp item or a dull item. Record your findings in Table 15.6.

4. Repeat the above maneuvers, this time on the left forehead. Record the results in Table 15.7.

5. Repeat the sharp and dull test again on the right cheek. Record the results in Table 15.8.

6. Repeat the test again on the left cheek. Record your findings in Table 15.9.

7. Repeat the test again on the right side of the jaw. Record your findings in Table 15.10.

8. Repeat one final time on the left side of the jaw and record your findings in Table 15.11.

9. Tests 4–9 test the function of sensory nerves in CN V. Were there any discrepancies? If so, were they more common on one side of the face or in a particular location?

_____

_____

_____

- **If the sensory function of CN V is healthy, the subject will be able to feel the cotton immediately and differentiate between a dull and sharp item. There will not be any large discrepancies between the different areas of the face/head.**

Table 15.6 Trigeminal Nerve Sensory Findings—Right Forehead	
Sensation Applied	**Subject's Response**

Table 15.7   Trigeminal Nerve Sensory Findings—Left Forehead

Sensation Applied	Subject's Response

Table 15.8   Trigeminal Nerve Sensory Findings—Right Cheek

Sensation Applied	Subject's Response

Table 15.9   Trigeminal Nerve Sensory Findings—Left Cheek

Sensation Applied	Subject's Response

Table 15.10 Trigeminal Nerve Sensory Findings—Right Jaw	
Sensation Applied	Subject's Response

Table 15.11 Trigeminal Nerve Sensory Findings—Left Jaw	
Sensation Applied	Subject's Response

Motor Assessment

1. Palpate the subject's temporal and masseter muscles and instruct the subject to clench the jaw as tightly as possible. Were there any differences in the strength of the muscle contractions between the right and left sides? If so, explain.

_____

_____

_____

● If the motor function of CN V is healthy, the strength of the muscle contraction should be approximately the same on both sides.

Cranial Nerve VII: Facial Nerve

1. Instruct the subject to look up and wrinkle his or her forehead. Place both hands on either side of the forehead and test the strength of the muscle by pulling down on the forehead. Is there any difference in the strength of the muscle on the right and left sides? If so, explain.

_____

_____

_____

2. Observe the subject performing the following movements. Look for any differences in muscle contraction between the right and left sides and record your findings.
   a. Eyes shut tight
   b. Frowning
   c. Showing upper teeth
   d. Exposing lower teeth
   e. Puffing out the cheeks

_____

_____

_____

_____

_____

_____

_____

● **If CN VII is healthy, the strength of the muscle contractions on both sides of the face should be approximately equal in both tests.**

Cranial Nerve VIII: Vestibulocochlear Nerve

1. Stand one to two feet to the right of the subject and instruct him or her to occlude their left ear by putting a finger in it and to turn the head to the left. Say that you are going to whisper a word or phrase that the subject should tell you when it can be heard.

2. Whisper a word or phrase to the subject, moving closer to the subject until he or she can hear you. Ask the subject to repeat the word or phrase you were whispering. Report your findings for the right ear:

_____

_____

3. Repeat, this time standing on the left side of the subject while the subject occludes the right ear and turns the head to the right. Record your findings for the left ear:

_____

_____

_____

4. Were there any differences in hearing between the right and left ear (i.e., were you about the same distance on both sides before the subject heard you)? If so, explain the difference.

_____

_____

_____

● **If CN VIII is healthy, the sound should be heard from approximately the same distance on both sides.**

Cranial Nerves IX and X: Glossopharyngeal Nerve and Vagus Nerve

1. Instruct the subject to speak (anything) and listen to the quality of the sound. Does it sound hoarse? Nasal? Report your findings below.

_____

_____

2. Tell the subject to open his or her mouth wide and say "ah." Observe the uvula (the structure that hangs down from the back of the mouth). Does the uvula remain at the midline? If not, where is it?

_____

_____

3. Repeat the above, this time watching for symmetry in the movement of the soft palate. Did both sides move symmetrically? If not, explain your observations.

_____

_____

_____

● If CN IX and X are healthy, the voice should not be hoarse or nasal (unless the subject has a cold!). The uvula should remain at the midline, and both sides of the soft palate should move symmetrically.

Cranial Nerve XI: Accessory Nerve

1. Place your hands on the subject's shoulders (you can either be facing each other or you can be behind the subject) and apply resistance. Tell the subject to move his or her shoulders up against the resistance. Is there any difference in the strength of the trapezius contractions on the right and left sides? If so, describe the differences.

_____

_____

_____

● If CN XI is healthy, the strength of the muscle contraction should be the same on both sides.

Cranial Nerve XII: Hypoglossal Nerve

1. Have the subject speak. Listen to the articulation of the words. Report your findings below.

_____

_____

2. Instruct the subject to stick out his or her tongue. Does the tongue move (deviate) in any way from the midline of the mouth? If so, describe the direction of the deviation.

_____

_____

● If CN XII is healthy, speech should be articulate and the tongue should be at the midline.

Cranial Nerve Assessment

Did the results of all of the tests come out as expected? If not, state the cranial nerve and describe the discrepancy.

_____

_____

_____

_____

Reflex Activity

This activity investigates two reflexes. The first is the patellar stretch reflex. This reflex is a spinal somatic reflex, which means that the information is integrated within the spinal cord (and is not controlled by the higher brain areas) and stimulates skeletal muscle. The second reflex involves reaction time, which is how long it takes to respond to a stimulus. In this reflex, higher brain levels are used to interpret the visual cues and elicit a motor response.

Activity Instructions

Follow the directions below to test the patellar stretch reflex and reaction times. Work with a partner, decide who will be the subject, and switch roles if time permits.

Patellar Stretch Reflex

1. Have your subject sit on the lab bench with legs dangling. Use the percussion hammer and gently hit the subject's patellar ligament. What reaction occurred? Was it fast or slow? Which muscle group contracted?

   _____

   _____

   _____

2. Tell the subject to do a wall squat (squat with the back to the wall) and hold it for as long as possible (until muscle fatigue occurs). Retest the patellar stretch reflex. How was it different from the above reaction?

   _____

   _____

   _____

Testing the Reaction-Time Reflex

1. Instruct the subject to stand facing you, with the dominant arm extended and the thumb and index finger extended (as if pinching something).

2. Hold a metric ruler vertically approximately 3 cm above the subject's hand. Tell the subject to catch the ruler as quickly as possible, using the thumb and index finger. Drop the ruler and record the distance at which the subject caught the ruler. Record the results in Table 15.12. Repeat five times.

3. How did reaction times change as the subject went through the trials?

_____

_____

_____

4. Pick a code word. Repeat the experiment above, but this time say a word each time you drop the ruler. The subject should catch the ruler only when the code word is stated; every time the ruler is released and a word other than the code word is stated, the ruler should drop to the floor. Record your results, as before, in Table 15.13.

5. How did reaction times compare with those from the first set of trials? Why do you think that change occurred? How many times did the subject catch the ruler when the code word was not stated?

_____

_____

_____

_____

6. Write a paragraph about this reflex loop, including the terms **eye, motor cortex, spinal cord, receptor, sensory neuron, motor neuron, skeletal muscle,** and **occipital lobe.** These words are not necessarily listed in the order in which you should use them in your paragraph.

_____

_____

_____

_____

_____

_____

_____

Table 15.12 Reaction Times — Control	
Trial Number	**Distance at Which Ruler Was Caught (cm)**

Table 15.13 Reaction Times — Variable	
Trial Number	**Distance at Which Ruler Was Caught (cm)**

Post-Lab Assessment

1. Name the cranial nerve that is responsible for hearing.

   _____

2. Name the cranial nerve that controls the trapezius.

   _____

3. Name the structures found in the diencephalon.

   _____

   _____

4. Compare the patellar reflex and the reaction time reflex that you tested in today's lab. How
   were they the same? How were they different?

   _____

   _____

   _____

   _____

5. Name the crack that separates the two cerebral hemispheres. Name the fold of dura mater
   located in this crack.

   _____

   _____

6. Name the space located between the pons and the cerebellum.

   _____

7. Name the modified blood vessels that produce and secrete CSF.

   _____

16

The Special Senses

Textbook Correlation: Chapter 9—Sensation: The Somatic and Special Senses

Details

Activities	Activity Objectives	Required Materials	Estimated Time
16-1: Eye Anatomy	Identify the structures of the eye.	• Eye model	20 min
16-2: Microscopic Eye Anatomy	Identify the microscopic structures of the eye.	• Stereoscope • Microscope • Eye slide	15 min
16-3: Sheep or Cow Eye Dissection	Identify the parts of a sheep or cow eye.	• Dissection tray • Scissors • Scalpel • Eye	15–20 min
16-4: Ear Anatomy	Identify the parts of the ear.	• Ear model • Labyrinth model (optional) • Cochlea model	30 min
16-5: Histology of the Cochlea	Identify the microscopic parts of the cochlea.	• Microscope • Cochlea slide	15 min
16-6: Weber Test	Assess and mimic conduction deafness.	• Tuning fork (500–1,000 Hz cycles/sec)	10 min
16-7: Romberg Test	Assess vestibular system damage.	• Chalkboard • Chalk	10 min
16-8: Taste and Smell	Determine the effect that smell has on taste.	• Blindfold • "Mystery Items"	20 min

Overview

Try this experiment: Stand on one foot and reach out to touch a particular spot on the wall. Easy, right? Next, spin around 20 times, close your eyes, and repeat the experiment. The simple task is no longer so simple, because you are interfering with the normal functioning of two special senses; vision and equilibrium (balance). Today's lab investigates the form and function of the organs responsible for vision and equilibrium: the eye and the ear (respectively). We will also examine another function of the ear—hearing.

Now try this experiment: close your eyes and ask someone (family member, roommate) to give you a food item. Try to guess the identity of the food item. It was probably harder than you thought! Today we will also investigate the fantastic world of taste as well as the effect that olfaction (smell) has on taste.

Safety note: At the beginning of today's lab activities, please notify your instructor if you have any food allergies.

Need to Know

- **Eye:** the organ that receives light waves and transduces (or changes the type of energy) the waves into electrical impulses that can then be transmitted to the brain via the optic nerve. The eye is composed of three layers (tunics) and the lens (not a layer):
  - **Fibrous tunic:** the most superficial layer of the eye, which is thick (fibrous) and protective. Includes the:
    - ○ **Sclera:** the white portion of the eye.
    - ○ **Cornea:** the bulging, transparent part of the fibrous tunic that helps focus the image on the retina.
  - **Lens:** transparent structure that also focuses the light waves on the retina. If the lens is structurally abnormal in shape or size, a person wears corrective lenses (glasses or contact lenses).
  - **Vascular tunic:** deep to the fibrous tunic; contains:
    - ○ **Choroid:** reddish-brown layer deep to the fibrous tunic; highly vascularized; supplies the other tunics with nutrients.
    - ○ **Iris:** anterior portion of the vascular tunic; the colorful part of the eye.
    - ○ **Ciliary body:** bulge of the choroid posterior and lateral to the iris; the **suspensory ligaments** extend from the ciliary body to the lens to suspend it and change the shape of the lens to bring an image into focus.
    - ○ **Pupil:** a hole located in the middle of the iris though which light passes; changes in pupil diameter vary the amount of light passing into the eye.
  - **Neural tunic (retina):** the deepest layer of the eye; contains:
    - ○ Three types of cells:
      - ■ **Photoreceptors:** Cones detect color and rods detect variations in light intensity. These cells transduce the incoming light waves into electrical impulses.
      - ■ **Bipolar cells:** receive electrical impulses from the photoreceptors and pass them on to the ganglion cells.
      - ■ **Ganglion cells:** the axons of these cells form the optic nerve.
    - ○ **Optic disc:** spot on the retina where the axons of ganglion cells cluster before exiting the eye as the optic nerve.
    - ○ **Macula lutea:** yellow dot located on the retina that is the center of focus; it contains the highest number of cones.
  - The eye contains chambers that contain humors (fluids).
    - ○ **Anterior chamber:** located between the cornea and lens; it contains aqueous humor.

○ **Posterior chamber:** located between the lens and the retina; it contains vitreous humor.
● **Ear:** the organ that transduces sound waves into electrical impulses for "hearing" and also maintains balance. It is divided into three areas:
  ● **External ear:** the outermost part of the ear:
    ○ **Pinna (auricle):** attached laterally to the head
    ○ **External auditory canal:** brings sound waves from the external environment to the middle ear
  ● **Middle ear:** chamber within the temporal bone which contains the:
    ○ **Tympanic membrane ("eardrum"):** a thin membrane that vibrates with incoming sound waves
    ○ **Ossicles:** the smallest bones of the body; they are the
      ▪ **Malleus:** attached to and receives sound waves from the tympanic membrane
      ▪ **Incus:** attached to and receives sound waves from the malleus
      ▪ **Stapes:** receives sound waves from the incus
    ○ **Oval window:** small, oval, flexible membrane that the stapes rests against
    ○ **Round window:** small, round, flexible membrane located inferior to the oval window
    ○ **Auditory tube:** connects the ear with the pharynx, allowing air to move in and out of the middle ear in order to equalize pressure with the atmosphere (prevents the tympanic membrane from perforating).
  ● **Inner ear:** space carved out of the temporal bone (bony labyrinth, filled with perilymph) containing a membranous labyrinth filled with endolymph.
    ○ **Cochlea:** snail shell–shaped structure that coils 2½ times and is responsible for converting sound waves into electrical impulses.
      ▪ **Cochlear duct:** membranous tube of the cochlea; it contains the **organ of Corti,** a tent-shaped structure whose hair cells convert the sound wave to an electrical signal; and the **tectorial membrane,** which extends from the top of the hair cells to the wall of the cochlea.
      ▪ **Vestibular duct:** space between the cochlear duct and the bony labyrinth; it opens up at the oval window.
      ▪ **Tympanic duct:** space between the cochlear duct and the bony labyrinth; it opens up at the round window.
      ▪ **Vestibular membrane:** thin membrane composed of simple squamous epithelium that separates the vestibular duct from the cochlear duct.
      ▪ **Basilar membrane:** thicker membrane that separates the cochlear duct from the tympanic duct.
    ○ **Vestibular apparatus:** a series of fluid-filled chambers that maintain equilibrium (balance):
      ▪ **Semicircular canals:** assess rotational acceleration
      ▪ **Otilith organs (utricle and saccule):** assess linear acceleration (including gravity)

Pre-Lab Activity

Students should complete this activity before completing the lab activities that follow.

1. List the tunics of the eye from deepest to most superficial.

   _____

   _____

2. Name the structure that separates the two chambers of the eye.

   _____

3. Label the accompanying illustration with the eye terms used in the "Need to Know" section and in the textbook.

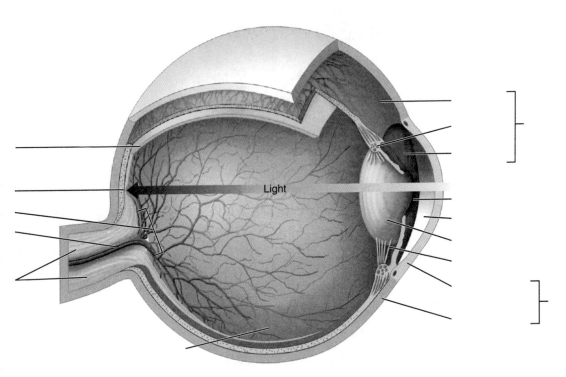

4. Name the structure in the inner ear that is responsible for transducing sound waves into electrical impulses.

_____

5. Label the accompanying illustration with the ear terms used in the "Need to Know" section.

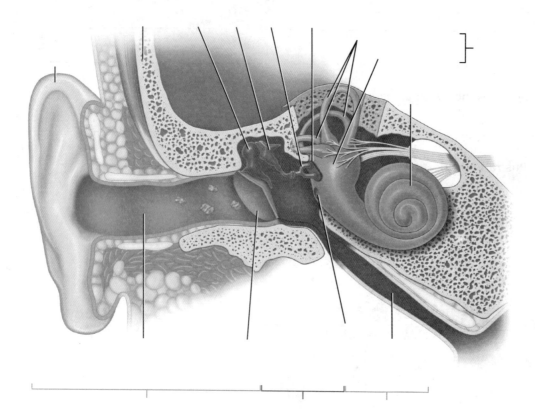

6. Label the accompanying illustration with the ear terms used in the "Need to Know" section.

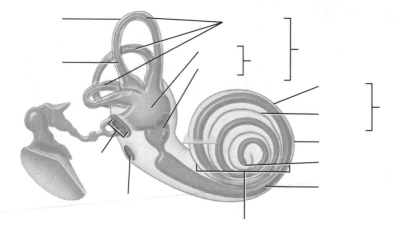

Eye Anatomy

Activity Instructions

On the eye model, identify the structures listed in the left-hand column of Table 16.1. As you identify each structure, write down the corresponding number in the right-hand column. You can use your pre-lab activity or Figures 9.15 to 9.17 of the textbook for reference.

Table 16.1 Eye Anatomy	
Structure	**Corresponding Number on Model**
Lacrimal gland	
Superior rectus	
Lateral rectus	
Medial rectus	
Superior oblique	
Inferior oblique	
Lens	
Sclera	
Cornea	
Choroid	

(continued)

Table 16.1 Eye Anatomy (continued)	
Structure	**Corresponding Number on Model**
Ciliary body	
Suspensory ligaments	
Iris	
Pupil	
Circular muscles	
Radial muscles	
Neural tunic (retina)	
Macula lutea	
Optic nerve	
Optic disc	
Anterior chamber (between cornea and lens) filled with aqueous humor	
Posterior chamber (between lens and retina) filled with vitreous humor	

Activity Questions

1. If the lacrimal gland is not present on the model, how can you distinguish between the medial and lateral rectus? Hint: look at the tendon of the superior oblique.

_____

_____

2. Does the eye contain more vitreous humor or aqueous humor? Explain your answer.

_____

_____

_____

3. Name the colored portion of the eye.

_____

4. Name the hole in the eye that can change in size to regulate the amount of light that hits the retina.

_____

5. Which group of eye muscles (extraocular or pupillary muscles) are somatic, or composed of skeletal muscle? How do you know?

_____

_____

6. What cranial nerve number is the optic nerve?

_____

7. Refer to Table 9.1 in your textbook. Look to the right of the room without moving your head. Which extraocular muscle moved your right eye? Which muscle moved your left eye?

_____

_____

8. Look up and to the left without moving your head. Which two extraocular muscles move the right eye? Which two extraocular muscles move the left eye?

_____

_____

Microscopic Eye Anatomy

Activity Instructions

1. Identify the following structures under the demo stereoscope. Draw, label, and describe your findings.
   - Lens
   - Fibrous tunic
     - Sclera
     - Cornea
   - Vascular tunic
     - Choroid
     - Ciliary body
     - Suspensory ligaments
     - Iris
       - Pupil
   - Neural tunic (retina)
   - Optic nerve
   - Optic disc
   - Anterior chamber (between the lens and the cornea)
   - Posterior chamber (between the lens and the retina)

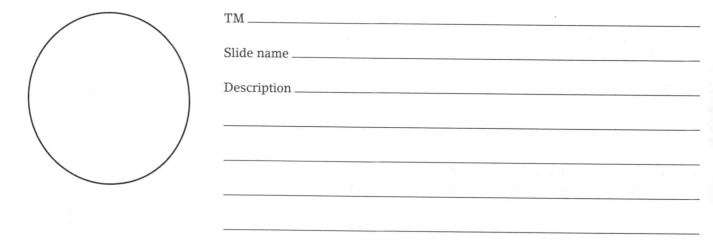

TM _____

Slide name _____

Description _____

_____

_____

_____

_____

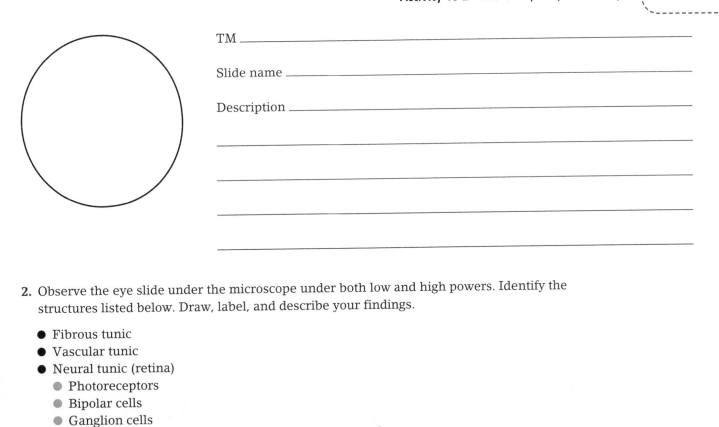

TM _____

Slide name _____

Description _____

_____

_____

_____

_____

2. Observe the eye slide under the microscope under both low and high powers. Identify the structures listed below. Draw, label, and describe your findings.

- Fibrous tunic
- Vascular tunic
- Neural tunic (retina)
  - Photoreceptors
  - Bipolar cells
  - Ganglion cells
- Axons of ganglion cells
- Optic nerve
- Optic disc

TM _____

Slide name _____

Description _____

_____

_____

_____

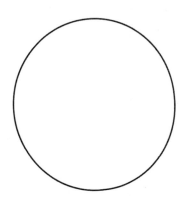

TM _____

Slide name _____

Description _____

_____

_____

Activity Questions

1. Name the two cell layers in the retina through which the light wave must pass before it reaches the photoreceptors.

  _____

2. In order, list the cells that are activated by the light ray.

  _____

3. Name the structures that project from the ciliary body and hold the lens in place.

  _____

Activity 16-3

Sheep or Cow Eye Dissection

Activity Instructions

1. Obtain a dissecting tray, scalpel, scissors, and one eye per group of four students.

2. Identify the following external structures:
   - Optic nerve
   - Sclera
   - Cornea
   - Iris

3. The eye might contain a large amount of adipose tissue. If it does, use the scissors to remove it.

4. Use the scalpel to perform a frontal section of the eye. Insert the scalpel approximately 1/4 in. posterior to the cornea. The sclera is very thick, so we recommend that you stick the point of the scalpel through the sclera and then work your way around the eye. **Safety note:** Remember, the eye contains fluid that has been enclosed in the eye. Use caution when cutting open the eye to prevent the fluid from spraying you and getting into your eyes. Your instructor may require you to wear safety goggles during this portion of the dissection.

5. Identify the following structures:
- Pupil
- Lens
- Vitreous humor (most likely spilled in the tray)
- Choroid
  - Tapetum lucidum
    - ○ This iridescent layer of the choroid is found in the eyes of many nocturnal vertebrates. It reflects light back on the retina in order to allow for greater night vision; however, the reflected light diminishes the sharpness of the image, making it more blurry.
    - ○ When you take a flash photo of a friend, the pupils don't have time to contract to limit the incoming light; therefore it is reflected off the reddish choroid. This bounce-back effect is "red eye." Now think about flash photos of cats or dogs. Those animals typically have "green eye" because the iridescent tapetum lucidum is reflected back.
- Retina

Activity 16-4

Ear Anatomy

Activity Instructions

On the ear models, identify the structures listed in the left-hand column of Table 16.2. As you identify each structure, write down the type of ear model and the corresponding number in the right-hand column. You can use your pre-lab activity or Figures 9.7 and 9.8 of your textbook for reference.

Table 16.2 Ear Anatomy		
Structure	**Model**	**Corresponding Number on the Model**
Pinna (auricle)		
External auditory canal		

(continued)

Table 16.2   Ear Anatomy (continued)

Structure	Model	Corresponding Number on the Model
Tympanic membrane		
Tympanic cavity containing the ossicles (malleus, incus, stapes)		
Oval window		
Round window		
Auditory tube		
Cochlea		
Cochlear duct		
Organ of Corti		
Tectorial membrane		
Vestibular membrane		
Basilar membrane		
Vestibular apparatus		
Three semicircular canals		
Otilith organs: utricle, saccule		
Vestibulocochlear nerve		

Activity Questions

1. Which two ducts does the vestibular membrane separate?

_____

2. Which membrane is found entirely within the cochlear duct?

_____

3. Is the cochlea responsible for maintaining equilibrium or for hearing?

_____

4. Name the tube in the ear that brings incoming sound waves to the tympanic membrane.

_____

5. Differentiate between the cochlea and the cochlear duct.

_____

_____

_____

_____

_____

6. Name the tube that originates at the round window.

_____

7. Which duct does not contain perilymph: the vestibular duct, the tympanic duct, or the cochlear duct? What fluid does it contain instead?

_____

8. Name the ear structure that can rupture with excessive pressure.

_____

9. List the three ossicles in the order that they conduct sound waves.

_____

Histology of the Cochlea

Activity Instructions

1. Identify the parts of the cochlea under low and high powers (the detail of the cochlear duct is best seen at high power). Draw, label, and describe your findings.
   - Cochlear duct
     - Organ of Corti
     - Hair cells
     - Tectorial membrane
   - Vestibular duct
   - Tympanic duct
   - Vestibular membrane
   - Basilar membrane

TM _____

Slide name _____

Description _____

_____

_____

_____

_____

TM _____

Slide name _____

Description _____

_____

_____

_____

Weber Test

There are two types of hearing loss:

- **Conduction** hearing loss: damage, blockage, or structural defects of the external or middle ear decrease the amount of sound waves reaching the cochlea.
- **Sensorineural** hearing loss: damage to the organ of Corti, (most common cause), vestibulo-cochlear nerve, or brain decreases sound wave transduction or nerve impulse conduction.

This test can detect the presence of both types of hearing loss; however, it can detect conduction hearing loss only if the hearing loss is unilateral (in one ear only). Bilateral conduction loss would involve equal hearing loss in both ears, so the result for this test would be normal.

Activity Instructions

1. Get a tuning fork (500 to 1,000 Hz cycles/sec). Choose a lab partner to be the subject. Gently strike the tuning fork against the desk so that soft sounds vibrate from the fork.

2. Ask the subject to close his or her eyes. Place the fork tines flat against your subject's forehead, right in the midline. Ask the subject where the sound is coming from (i.e., in which ear the sound is the loudest). Record the subject's response below.

_____

3. Switch roles and become the subject.

Activity Questions

1. Did both you and your subject respond that the sound came from the midline? If not, what was the response?

_____

2. In unilateral conduction deafness the sound is loudest in the affected ear. The bones of the skull conduct most of the sound directly to the inner ear, bypassing the external and middle ear structures, and the conduction defect blocks ambient room noises that would otherwise drown out the tuning fork. To see the effects of conduction deafness, plug your ear with your finger and repeat the test. Ask your lab partner to do the same. Which ear heard the sound best? Explain your answer.

_____

_____

_____

3. The opposite is true if there is sensorineural deafness in one ear; the sound is lowest in the affected ear (loudest in the unaffected ear). Explain why based on your understanding of the mechanics of hearing.

_____

_____

_____

Activity 16-7

Romberg Test

This test assesses the functioning of the vestibular system in maintaining balance.

Activity Instructions

1. Instruct your subject to stand in front of the chalk (or white) board, facing you with feet together and arms at the sides.

2. Draw two lines on the board, outlining the subject's torso. The lines will serve as reference marks.

3. Tell the subject to stand there, in that position, for 1 minute. Observe the subject for swaying. Did the subject sway slightly or considerably?

_____

4. Repeat the instructions above, but this time instruct the subject to keep his or her eyes closed for 1 minute. Did the subject sway slightly more or considerably more than with the eyes open?

_____

Activity Questions

1. Why do you think that there was more swaying when the subject's eyes were closed?

2. How do you think the results would have been different if there were damage to the vestibular system?

Activity 16-8

Taste and Smell

Activity Instructions

Be sure to choose a subject who does not have a cold or nasal congestion.

1. Blindfold your subject and place a clothespin (or other object) over the nose, closing off the nares (nostrils).

2. Feed the subject mystery item #1 by placing it directly in the mouth. For each mystery item, ask the following questions and fill in the corresponding columns in Table 16.3:
   • "Describe the texture of the item."
   • "Describe the primary taste (sour, salty, sweet, bitter, unami) of the item." Remind students that "unami" means meaty or savory in Japanese.
   • "Based on your conclusions, what do you think you just consumed?"

3. Repeat step 2 for the different mystery items.

4. Keep the blindfold on the subject but remove the nose clips and repeat the test. Record the responses in Table 16.4.

5. Once the data have been collected, ask the instructor for the key to the mystery results.

Table 16.3 "No Smell" Taste Data

Mystery Item Number	Texture	Primary Taste	Subject's Conclusion
1			
2			
3			
4			
5			
6			
7			

Table 16.4 "Smell" Taste Data

Mystery Item Number	Texture	Primary Taste	Subject's Conclusion
1			
2			
3			
4			
5			
6			
7			

Activity Questions

1. Did the subject get any mystery items correct while wearing the nose pin? If so, was there a common primary taste that the subject identified correctly?

_____

_____

_____

_____

2. Did the subject get more mystery items correct when the nose pin was removed? Why?

_____

_____

_____

3. Smoking interferes with both taste and olfaction by decreasing (and overriding) the functioning of the taste buds, the gustatory center in the brain, and the epithelium in the nasal cavity. How do you think taste and olfaction change when a person stops smoking?

_____

_____

_____

Post-Lab Assessment

1. Match the following structures with correct tunic of the eye:

   a. Fibrous tunic
   b. Neural tunic
   c. Vascular tunic

   _____ Choroid

   _____ Ciliary body

   _____ Cornea

   _____ Iris

   _____ Macula lutea

   _____ Optic disc

   _____ Retina

   _____ Rods

   _____ Sclera

2. Match the following structures with the location in the ear:

   a. Cochlea
   b. External ear
   c. Middle ear
   d. Vestibular apparatus

   _____ Auditory tube

   _____ Basilar membrane

   _____ Cochlear duct

   _____ External auditory canal

   _____ Incus

   _____ Malleus

   _____ Semicircular canals

   _____ Stapes

   _____ Tympanic duct

   _____ Tympanic membrane

   _____ Vestibular duct

   _____ Vestibular membrane

3. Jung finally saved enough money to buy a new Mp3 player. He listened to it constantly (walking around campus, doing chores, exercising, studying) at a relatively high volume, using the ear buds that came with the device. Several years later, he was doing hearing tests with his partner in an anatomy lab. To his chagrin, he was not hearing many of the sounds that he was supposed to be hearing. Jung made an appointment with his physician, who ran several hearing tests. The physician concluded that Jung, only 24 years old, suffered from partial hearing loss due to the frequent use of and high volume of his Mp3 player. What type of hearing loss do you think was most prominent in Jung? Explain your answer.

_____

_____

_____

_____

_____

4. In the smell-versus-taste test, why was it important to choose a subject that did not have a cold or nasal congestion?

_____

_____

_____

17

Blood

Textbook Correlation: Chapter 10—Blood

Details

Activities	Activity Objectives	Required Materials	Estimated Time
17-1: Blood Cell Identification	Identify the types of blood cells; differentiate between the granulocytes and the agranulocytes	● Microscope ● Blood smear slide	25 min
17-2: Hematocrit	Centrifuge simulated blood to obtain a hematocrit value	● Simulated blood ● Microhematocrit capillary tubes ● Sealing clay ● Centrifuge	15 min
17-3: Blood Typing	Perform a blood typing exercise and interpret the results	● Simulated blood kit ● Plastic toothpicks	20–25 min
17-4: Case Studies	Apply your knowledge of blood types and transfusions in a series of case studies		30 min

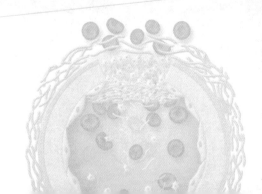

Overview

Jason was walking home from the basketball courts when a group of young males approached him and demanded his wallet. Jason tried to flee but his assailants caught up to him and pinned him to the ground. While one stole his wallet, another stabbed him several times and he lost consciousness. Luckily, a passerby found him and called 911; he was then rushed to the hospital. "Quick!! The patient is crashing! He needs a blood transfusion immediately!" The ER nurse set up the transfusion and, within minutes, donor blood was circulating in Jason's blood vessels, replacing the blood he'd lost and maintaining his life while the team prepared him for emergency surgery.

Think about it: Jason arrived in the ER in critical condition, so there was no time to test his blood type. Given this, what type of blood did the nurse transfuse? How can you be certain?

Need to Know

- Blood is a type of connective tissue because it is derived from mesenchyme and contains an extracellular matrix and cells.

- **Extracellular matrix:**
  - **Plasma:** the liquid portion of blood; a watery fluid containing electrolytes, glucose, amino acids, and various other solutes

- **Cells:**
  - **Erythrocytes** (or red blood cells—RBCs): red, biconcave discs approximately 7 to 8 μm in diameter
    - Contain **hemoglobin,** the protein that transports oxygen in blood
  - **Leukocytes** (white blood cells—WBCs):
    - **Granulocytes:** contain cytoplasmic granules
      - **Neutrophils:** most populous of the WBCs; granules stain pink to purple and nucleus contains many lobes.
      - **Eosinophils:** granules stain brick red and nucleus is shaped like a shallow U.
      - Both of the above are slightly larger than an erythrocyte.
      - **Basophils:** slightly smaller than an erythrocyte; the cytosol is filled with dark bluish-purple staining granules that typically occlude the nucleus.
    - **Agranulocytes:** do not contain cytoplasmic granules; both cells contain a large nucleus that stains dark purple and takes over most of the cytoplasm.
      - **Lymphocytes:** approximately the same size as a basophil
      - **Monocyte:** approximately twice the size of an erythrocyte
  - **Platelets:** very small cell fragments that resembles debris on the slide
  - **Hematocrit:** percentage of whole blood volume occupied by erythrocytes
    - Obtained using a **centrifuge** that spins the blood to separate the components; erythrocytes sink to the bottom.
    - **Male value:** 47% (±5%)
    - **Female value:** 42% (±5%)

- **Blood typing:** process that determines the *antigens* present on an individual's RBCs
  - **Antigen:** any substance capable of inducing an immune reaction.
  - **Antibodies:** proteins that attack non-self (foreign) antigens.
  - Mixing different blood types results in blood cell clumping (agglutination).

- **ABO antigen system (see Table 17.1, below):**
  - ○ Determined by the presence or absence of type A and type B antigens on RBC surfaces.
  - ○ Genetically determined.
  - ○ Each person's plasma contains antibodies against antigens NOT present on his or her RBCs.
- **Rh (Rh D) antigen system**
  - ○ RBCs either have the antigen (Rh positive) or do not have the antigen (Rh negative).
  - ○ **Anti–Rh D antibodies:**
    - ■ Only produced after Rh negative blood is exposed to Rh positive blood.
    - ■ Agglutination occurs the second time Rh positive blood is encountered.

Table 17.1   ABO Blood Types

Blood Type	Antigen on RBCs	Antibody in Plasma
A	A	B
B	B	A
AB	A and B	None
O	None	A, B

Pre-Lab Activity

Students should complete this activity before completing the lab activities that follow.

1. Color the following pictures according to the color scheme used in Table 10.1 of your textbook. Name each cell.

  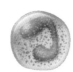

2. Name the antigen(s) found on type A erythrocytes. Name the antibodies (if any) found in the plasma.

_____

3. Name the antigen(s) found on type AB erythrocytes. Name the antibodies (if any) found in the plasma.

_____

4. Does an Rh negative individual possess Rh antigens on the erythrocytes?

_____

5. Who would produce anti-Rh antibodies, and when?

_____

Blood Cell Identification

Activity Instructions

1. Identify the following microscopic blood cells (under the high-power and oil-immersion lenses) listed below. Draw, label, and describe your findings.
   - Erythrocytes
   - Leukocytes
     - Neutrophils
     - Eosinophils
     - Basophils
     - Monocytes
     - Lymphocytes
   - Platelets (thrombocytes)

TM _____

Slide name _____

Description _____

_____

_____

_____

_____

TM _____

Slide name _____

Description _____

_____

_____

_____

TM _____

Slide name _____

Description _____

_____

_____

_____

_____

TM _____

Slide name _____

Description _____

_____

_____

_____

_____

TM _____

Slide name _____

Description _____

_____

_____

_____

_____

TM _____

Slide name _____

Description _____

_____

_____

_____

_____

Activity Questions

1. How do neutrophils resemble eosinophils under the microscope? What is different about their appearance?

_____

_____

_____

_____

2. How do basophils and lymphocytes resemble one another microscopically? How can you tell the difference between the two cells?

_____

_____

_____

_____

3. How are monocytes best distinguished from lymphocytes?

_____

_____

4. How does the appearance of granulocytes differ from that of agranulocytes?

_____

_____

_____

5. **Critical Thinking:** One of the many jobs of investigators (forensic scientists) at crime scenes is to collect DNA evidence by obtaining blood samples. Erythrocytes do not have a nucleus, therefore no DNA … so what are the forensic scientists analyzing in the blood sample in order to match DNA? Explain your answer.

_____

_____

_____

_____

Activity 17-2

Hematocrit

Activity Instructions

1. Obtain a vial of simulated blood and a microhematocrit capillary tube. Fill the tube approximately ¾ full (to the black line) with the simulated blood and seal the end of the tube with sealing clay.

2. Place the tube in the centrifuge machine with the seal facing the bottom of the machine (black line facing superior). Many centrifuge machines must be balanced, which means that if you place the tube at the 12 o'clock position, there must be another tube, equally full, at the 6 o'clock position in the machine.

3. Turn on the machine and centrifuge the blood for 3 to 5 minutes.

4. Remove hematocrit sample from the machine and get a small metric ruler. Place the hematocrit sample on a piece of white paper.

Activity Questions

1. Which component of the blood is located in the lowest part of the tube (on top of the sealing clay)? Why?

_____

_____

_____

2. Measure the height of erythrocytes in the tube. Record your answer using metric units.

_____

3. Measure and record (in metric units) the total height of the blood column.

_____

4. Calculate the hematocrit for your sample by dividing the total height by the erythrocyte height, and record it below.

_____

5. Is the value within normal range? If not, is the value close to the normal value or far from the norm?

_____

_____

_____

6. How do you think that the speed of the flow of blood would be affected if the hematocrit value increased substantially?

_____

_____

_____

Blood Typing

Activity Instructions

Experimental Setup

1. Obtain one simulated blood kit, four blood typing trays, and six plastic toothpicks.

2. Place the blood typing trays on a piece of paper (white unlined paper is best), one in each of the four corners.
   - Label the paper next to the tray in the **upper left** "Mr. Jones."
   - Label the paper next to the tray in the **upper right** "Mr. Smith."
   - Label the paper next to the tray in the **lower left** "Mr. Green,"
   - Label the paper next to the tray in the **lower right** "Ms. Brown."

3. Get the bottle of blood labeled "Mr. Jones" and shake it. Place several drops of the simulated blood in each well of Mr. Jones's tray (the wells are labeled "A," "B," and "Rh"). Do not completely fill or overfill the wells.

4. Obtain the bottle marked "Simulated Anti-A Serum" and place several drops in the well labeled "A." This bottle contains A antibodies. Repeat step 4 but put the Anti-B serum (containing B antibodies) in the B well and the Anti-Rh serum (with anti-Rh antibodies) in the Rh well.

5. Use one end of a toothpick to lightly swirl the blood around in well A (do not scrape the bottom of the tray). Use the other end of the toothpick to swirl the contents of well B. Use a different toothpick to swirl the contents in the Rh well. Be sure to use different ends of toothpicks for each well in order to prevent cross-contamination.

6. Repeat steps 3 to 5 for each of the other "people."

7. Allow each tray to sit for approximately 10 to 15 minutes before you read the results.

Activity Questions

Results

1. In the drawing below, label each tray with one of these names: Jones, Smith, Green, and Brown. Look for agglutination in the wells (A, B, Rh) for each person that you prepared. If agglutination has occurred, you will see crystal lattice structures that look like small cracks in glass, or fine hairs. Fill in the well circles in the figure for each well in which agglutination has occurred. Leave the other circles blank.

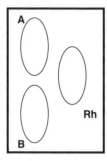 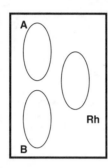 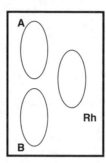 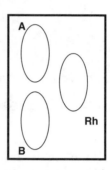

2. How would the wells appear in a type O⁺ individual? Why? Explain your results.

_____

_____

_____

_____

_____

3. Refer to your well plate drawings above and interpret your results. Fill in Table 17.2. Put a check mark in each box (for the specific individual) in which agglutination was observed. In the last column, write the blood type for the individual. Recall that agglutination (clumping) occurs if the RBCs have the antigens recognized by the specific antiserum added to the well.

4. Is anyone a universal donor? A universal recipient?

_____

_____

5. Check your answers with the instructor before moving on to the next activity. Correct any mistakes that you made in the boxes below.

Table 17.2 Blood Typing Results				
Subject's Name	A Well	B Well	Rh Well	Blood Type
Mr. Smith				
Mr. Jones				
Ms. Brown				
Mr. Green				

Activity 17-4

Case Studies

Activity Instructions

Use the correct results from Activity 17-3 to answer the following case study questions based on the "patients." Consult the "Need to Know" section when necessary.

Ms. Brown

Ms. Brown is a 48-year-old mother of two grown children. She was admitted into the hospital with major internal bleeding after a car accident. The following is her history.

1. Ms. Brown was pregnant 20 years ago with an Rh-positive fetus. Prior to that pregnancy, she had never had a blood transfusion. Were there any complications due to the mismatched Rh factor during that pregnancy? Explain your answer.

_____

_____

_____

_____

2. The labor and delivery nurse at her first pregnancy quickly scanned Ms. Brown's file and missed the fact that her blood type was O negative, so Ms. Brown was never given the RhoGAM shot after delivery and she was exposed to a small amount of the placental blood. The RhoGAM shot prevents sensitization of Rh-negative blood after the delivery of an Rh-positive baby. What begins to happen in Ms. Brown's body? Is it life-threatening at this stage? Explain why or why not.

_____

_____

_____

_____

3. Ms. Brown became pregnant again a few years later, again with an Rh-positive fetus, and the fetus's life was at risk. Why? Explain. (Hint: Some antibodies pass from maternal blood into fetal blood through the placenta.)

_____

_____

_____

_____

Fortunately, this issue was detected very early in her pregnancy and the hematologist (blood specialist) was able to save the fetus by performing intrauterine blood transfusions.

Now we are up to present and Ms. Brown is in the hospital…

4. En route to the hospital, the paramedic inserted an IV line filled with saline solution and plasma expanders in order to somewhat increase Ms. Brown's blood volume (and blood pressure). Upon arrival at the hospital, her blood was quickly typed and she was given a blood transfusion. For each blood type below, determine if it would have been an adequate match for Ms. Brown and explain why or why not.

a. O^+:

_____

_____

b. AB^-:

_____

_____

c. B⁻:

_____

_____

d. O⁻:

_____

_____

Mr. Green and Mr. Smith

Forensic scientists were called to a brutal crime scene; there was blood splatter everywhere and two victims, Mr. Green and Mr. Smith, were found dead. One person was holding a bloody lead pipe and the other held a bloody knife. Pictures of the crime scene were taken and evidence was collected. After interviewing several friends of both victims, it was determined that this was a murder scene in which one person murdered the other; then the murderer died either from his own injuries or because he was killed by another person who fled the scene.

1. Forensics discovered that the person holding the handle of the bloody knife had type A-positive blood. Refer to your table from Activity 3. Who was holding the knife?

_____

2. Blood of two types was found on the knife and lead pipe, meaning that both victims touched the weapons at some point during their struggle. Mr. Green was found with a large number of defensive stab wounds on his body as well as a severed femoral artery and several deep punctures to the chest. The blood evidence on the knife was consistent with the wounds because type AB-positive blood was found on the blade. Refer to your table from Activity 3. Based on the evidence, who do you think was killed first? Why?

_____

_____

_____

_____

3. However, type B-positive blood was also found on the lead pipe. Based on the evidence, do you think that another person was involved in the crime? Refer to your table from Activity 3. Why or why not? Explain your answer.

_____

_____

_____

_____

Mr. Jones

A 7.2 earthquake rumbled and shook southern Missouri. Many of the structures are very old and not retrograded to earthquake standards, despite the strong fault line below the ground. Mr. Jones was at work in an old, historic brick building when the earthquake struck and the building crumbled. He was stuck beneath much of the rubble. Several volunteer searchers found Mr. Jones two days later; he was confused and had lost a fairly substantial amount of blood. The rescuers took Mr. Jones to the field triage center, where he was quickly assessed by a team of trauma nurses and a physician; his blood type was also taken and recorded. (See the table in Activity 3.) The nurses searched the available blood supplies and all that they could locate was B-positive blood.

1. The medical staff then asked Mr. Jones a very important question. What do you think that the question was, based on his blood type and the blood type that the staff could provide for him? Why is that question important?

   _____

   _____

2. The team administered the blood to Mr. Jones. What precaution must he take in the future if he were to need another transfusion? Why?

   _____

   _____

   _____

   _____

Post-Lab Assessment

1. Name the three types of granulocytes.

   _____

2. Name the smallest agranulocyte.

   _____

3. A blood test is performed on a person who is found to be AB negative. In which wells will agglutination occur?

   _____

4. Name all of the blood types that a B-positive individual can receive.

   _____

18

Heart and Blood Vessel Anatomy

Textbook Correlation: Chapter 11—The Cardiovascular System

Details

Activities	Activity Objectives	Required Materials	Estimated Time
18-1: The Heart and Great Vessels	Identify the regions, walls, chambers, vessels, valves, and other structures of the heart	● Heart models	25–30 min
18-2: Sheep Heart Dissection	Identify the membranes, regions, walls, chambers, vessels and valves of the sheep heart	● Sheep heart ● Dissecting tray/pan ● Scalpel ● Scissors ● Probe	30–40 min
18-3: Blood Vessel Histology	Differentiate between an artery and vein microscopically; identify the tunics of the vessels; differentiate between the thickness of the tunicae in an artery versus a vein	● Microscope ● Artery and vein slide	15 min
18-4: Blood Vessel Identification	Identify various blood vessels of the body	● Torso model	45 min

Details *(Continued)*

Activities	Activity Objectives	Required Materials	Estimated Time
18-5: Modeling of the Abdominal Aorta	Model and identify the branches of the abdominal aorta	● Styrofoam cylinder ● Pipe cleaners: orange, green, purple, pink, yellow, blue, and white	20 min
18-6: Blood Vessel Mapping	Identify the major blood vessels of the body by drawing them	● Bone-mapping body outline (from Activity 11.2) ● Red marker ● Blue marker ● Purple marker	40 min

Overview

The heart is commonly used as a symbol of love and devotion. As children, we decorated paper hearts for our parents on Valentine's day; as adults, we give cards and balloons that are heart-shaped, or type a <3 code for the heart symbol to indicate our affection. We now know that it is the brain, not the heart, that controls emotions. However, the heart can respond to those emotions with a change in the rate of its beat!

The heart is a muscular pump that propels blood through the blood vessels, which are the closed tubes that transport the blood throughout the body. Today's lab will focus on studying the anatomy of the heart and the location of the blood vessels. The next lab period will focus on the physiology of the cardiovascular system. To see more dissection images, visit the text's online site and view the Dissection Atlas.

Need to Know

- ● **Heart**
  - ● Medial to the lungs, superior to the diaphragm, and anterior to the thoracic vertebrae
    - ○ **Base:** the "base" for the great vessels located superiorly
    - ○ **Apex:** the tip, located inferiorly
    - ○ **Coronary circulation:** supplies oxygen-rich blood to the heart muscle and carries away oxygen-poor blood
  - ● **Heart coverings:**
    - ○ **Fibrous pericardium:** the superficial, tough membrane that encloses the heart in a "pouch"
    - ○ **Serous pericardium:** a thin serous membrane composed of two layers
      - ■ **Parietal pericardium:** outer layer attached to the fibrous pericardium
      - ■ **Visceral pericardium:** inner layer attached to the heart wall
      - ■ Pericardial space: virtual fluid-filled space separating the two serous layers
  - ● **Heart wall layers:**
    - ○ **Epicardium:** the most superficial layer of the heart wall; it is called the visceral pericardium when referred to as a membrane.
    - ○ **Myocardium:** the thick, middle muscular layer.
    - ○ **Endocardium:** the innermost layer lining the heart chambers.

- **Heart chambers:**
  - ○ Right and left **atria:** the smaller, superior chambers that receive blood from veins.
  - ○ Right and left **ventricles:** the larger inferior chambers that propel blood into arteries; the large **interventricular** septum separates the two chambers.
- **Great vessels:** large vessels directly connected to the heart
  - ○ **Superior vena cava:** drains oxygen-poor blood from the head and upper limbs into the right atrium
  - ○ **Inferior vena cava:** brings oxygen-poor blood from the trunk and lower limbs into the right atrium
  - ○ **Pulmonary trunk:**
    - ■ Most medial and anterior vessel on the base of the heart
    - ■ Carries oxygen-poor blood from the right ventricle
    - ■ Splits into the right and left **pulmonary arteries** that carry blood to the lungs
  - ○ **Pulmonary veins:** located on the lateral sides of the atria; bring oxygen-rich blood from the lungs to the left atrium
  - ○ **Aorta:** located between the superior vena cava and the pulmonary trunk; carries oxygenated blood from the left ventricle to the systemic arteries
- Contains four **valves:**
  - ○ Two atrioventricular valves
    - ■ Separate atria from ventricles
    - ■ Prevent blood backflow into the atria when the ventricles contract
    - ■ Strengthened by fibrous cords called **chordae tendineae** embedded in the **papillary muscle** (muscle extension in the ventricle)
    - ■ **Right atrioventricular (tricuspid) valve** has three cusps
    - ■ **Left atrioventricular (mitral) valve** has two cusps
  - ○ Two semilunar valves
    - ■ Separate ventricles from major arteries
    - ■ Prevent blood backflow into ventricles when the ventricles relax
    - ■ **Pulmonary valve:** located between the right ventricle and the pulmonary trunk
    - ■ **Aortic valve:** located between the left ventricle and the aorta

- **Blood vessels:** transport blood throughout the body
  - **Tunics:** layers of the blood vessel wall
    - ○ **Tunica externa:** outermost layer, composed of collagen and elastic fibers
    - ○ **Tunica media:** middle layer, composed of smooth muscle
    - ○ **Tunica interna:** deepest layer, composed of endothelium, which allows for a smooth surface for uninterrupted blood flow
  - **Arteries:** carry blood away from the heart
    - ○ Need thicker walls to withstand high pressure
    - ○ **Pulmonary arteries:** carry oxygen-poor blood from the right ventricle to the lungs
    - ○ **Systemic arteries:** distribute oxygen and nutrient-rich blood to the cells of the body
  - **Capillaries:** very thin blood vessels responsible for gas exchange
    - ○ **Pulmonary capillaries:** pick up oxygen and drop off carbon dioxide in lungs
    - ○ **Systemic capillaries:** drop off oxygen and pick up carbon dioxide in tissues
  - **Veins:** carry blood toward the heart
    - ○ Low-pressure, thin-walled vessels
    - ○ **Pulmonary veins:** bring oxygen-rich blood back to the left atrium
    - ○ **Systemic veins:** bring oxygen-poor blood back to the right atrium

Pre-Lab Activity

Students should complete this activity before completing the lab activities that follow.

1. Describe the location of the heart in the body.

_____

_____

_____

_____

2. Label the following picture with the following terms (some terms may be used more than once). Write the names of the heart chambers directly on the figures.
   - Anterior interventricular artery
   - Circumflex artery
   - Coronary sinus
   - Left atrium
   - Left coronary artery
   - Left ventricle
   - Posterior interventricular artery
   - Right atrium
   - Right coronary artery
   - Right marginal artery
   - Right ventricle

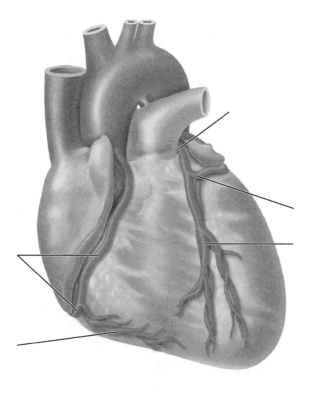
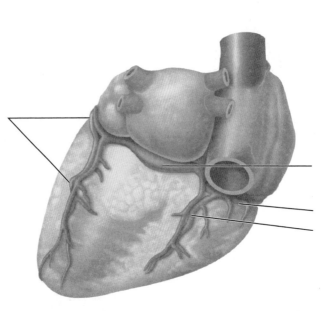

3. Label the four chambers on the picture below (draw your own leader lines). Color the picture using the colors listed below:
   - Aorta: red
   - Pulmonary trunk: light blue
   - Superior and inferior venae cavae: dark blue
   - Pulmonary veins: pink
   - Papillary muscles: orange
   - Right atrioventricular valve (tricuspid valve): brown
   - Left atrioventricular valve (mitral valve): green
   - Chordae tendineae: yellow
   - Interventricular septum: purple

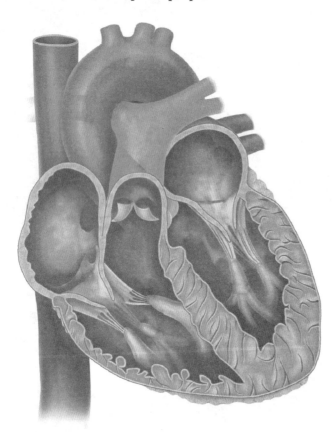

4. Use a black marker to draw arrows showing the correct sequence of blood flow through the heart on the diagram that you colored above.

5. There are two circulations through the heart: the **pulmonary circulation,** which brings blood to and from the lungs, and the **systemic circulation,** which brings blood to and from the rest of the body. Based on the description in the "Need to Know" section, which great vessels are part of the pulmonary circulation? Which vessels are part of the systemic circulation?

Pulmonary circulation:

_____

_____

_____

_____

Systemic circulation:

_____

_____

_____

6. List the tunics of a blood vessel from superficial to deep.

_____

7. Distinguish between an artery and a vein. Describe one structural difference and one functional difference.

_____

_____

_____

8. True or false: All arteries carry oxygen-rich blood and all veins carry oxygen-poor blood.

_____

The Heart and Great Vessels

Activity Instructions

On the heart model, identify the structures listed in the left-hand column of Table 18.1 below. As you identify each structure, write down the corresponding number in the right-hand column.

Table 18.1	
Structure	**Corresponding Number on Model**
Apex	
Base	
Epicardium (visceral pericardium when referring to it as a membrane)	
Myocardium	
Endocardium	
Right atrium	
Fossa ovalis	
Opening of coronary sinus	
Left atrium	
Right ventricle	
Left ventricle	
Interatrial septum	
Ascending aorta	
Pulmonary trunk	
Pulmonary arteries (right and left)	
Superior vena cava	
Inferior vena cava	

(continued)

Table 18.1 (continued)

Structure	Corresponding Number on Model
Pulmonary veins (right and left)	
Tricuspid valve (right atrioventricular valve)	
Mitral valve (left atrioventricular valve)	
Chordae tendineae	
Papillary muscles	
Aortic valve	
Pulmonary valve	
Coronary artery (right and left)	
Right marginal artery	
Circumflex artery	
Anterior interventricular artery	
Posterior interventricular artery	
Coronary sinus	

Activity Questions

1. Name the receiving chambers of the heart.

2. What is the alternate name for the right atrioventricular valve?

3. The coronary sinus returns the oxygen-poor blood into the _____ (name of chamber).

4. Where does blood go when the left ventricle contracts? Name the valve that blood passes through and the vessel that it enters.

5. Name the two great vessels that return oxygen-poor blood to the right atrium.

Sheep's Heart Dissection

Activity Instructions

External Anatomy

1. Obtain a dissecting tray, scalpel, scissors, probe, and sheep's heart (one per group of four students).

2. Follow steps 3 and 4 if the heart has the fibrous pericardium. If it does not, go directly to step 5.

3. Use the scissors to cut a slit through the fibrous pericardium and identify the following membranes:
    - Fibrous pericardium
    - Parietal pericardium
    - Visceral pericardium

4. Use the scissors to remove the thick pericardial membrane from the heart. Do not cut off any vessels.

5. Use the scissors to cut off the adipose tissue surrounding the heart. Be careful to avoid cutting off any vessels. You can come back and clean up the fat around the vessels later.
    Safety note: Be careful when handling the adipose tissue, because it tends to make your gloves and tray slippery. You may have to change your gloves after removing the adipose tissue so that the scalpel does not slip and cut you later.

6. Identify the **base** region and the **apex** region.

7. Place the heart on the tray ventral side up and you should see a dark-colored flap on your left side (the right side of the heart). That is the wall of the **right atrium.**

8. Find the opening at the top of the right atrium and insert your probe into the opening. That is the **superior vena cava.**

9. Find an opening that is inferior and slightly to the left of the superior vena cava and insert your probe. That is the **inferior vena cava.**

10. Look at the posterior side of the wall of the right atrium and you should see two small openings. Those are the **pulmonary veins.**

11. Look medially for the vessel that is most anterior and stick your probe through the opening. That is the **pulmonary trunk.**

12. Locate for the vessel that is between the pulmonary trunk and the superior vena cava. That is the **aorta.**

Internal Anatomy

1. Locate the superior vena cava again. Use your scalpel and make an incision from the superior vena cava to the apex of the heart, cutting through the wall of the right atrium and right ventricle.

2. Pull the two sides apart and locate the following structures:
   - Epicardium
   - Myocardium
   - Endocardium
   - Tricuspid valve
   - Chordae tendineae
   - Papillary muscles

3. Locate the pulmonary trunk and stick your probe through the opening. You should see the probe enter the **right ventricle.**

4. Use your scalpel and make an incision down the wall of the pulmonary trunk and look inside the vessel. You should be able to see the **pulmonary valve.**

5. Locate the base of the aorta again. Insert your scalpel through the wall of the left atrium and continue cutting inferiorly through the wall of the left ventricle until you get to the apex.

6. Open the newly created flap and identify the following walls and structures:
   - Epicardium
   - Myocardium
   - Endocardium
   - Mitral valve
   - Chordae tendineae
   - Papillary muscle

7. Stick your probe through the aorta and observe the probe entering the **left ventricle.**

8. Make an incision through the wall of the aorta and locate the **aortic semilunar valve.**

Activity Questions

1. Which ventricle has a thicker myocardium? Why?

_____

_____

_____

2. Describe the location of the pulmonary veins. Why does that location make sense? (Hint: Explain in terms of blood flow).

_____

_____

3. Describe the structural relationships between the papillary muscles, the atrioventricular valves, and the chordae tendineae.

_____

_____

Blood Vessel Histology

Activity Instructions

1. Obtain a slide that contains an artery and a vein. Look at your slide under scanning power and differentiate between an **artery** and a **vein.** Answer Activity Question 1.

2. Increase to low power and identify the following tunics (walls) of the artery. Draw and describe your findings below and answer Activity Question 2.
   - Tunica interna
   - Tunica media
   - Tunica externa

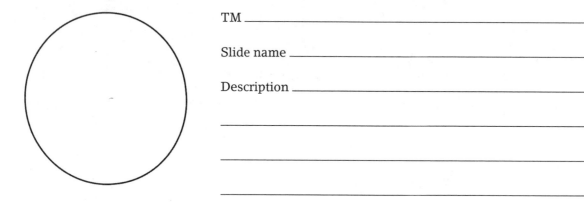

TM _____

Slide name _____

Description _____

_____

_____

_____

_____

3. Identify the tunics of the vein. Draw and describe your findings and answer the rest of the activity questions.
   - Tunica interna
   - Tunica media
   - Tunica externa

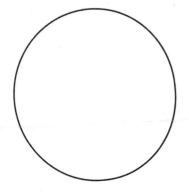

TM _____

Slide name _____

Description _____

_____

_____

_____

Activity Questions

1. How does the shape and size of the lumen differ between an artery and a vein?

_____

_____

_____

2. Which tunic is the thickest in the artery? Which is the thinnest?

_____

3. Which tunic is thickest in the vein? Which is the thinnest?

_____

4. How does the tunica media compare in the artery and vein?

_____

_____

_____

5. Name the kind of tissue that makes up the tunica media.

_____

6. **Critical Thinking:** The tissue that makes up the tunica interna is called the **endothelium** and is made up of a single layer of flat cells. What specific type of tissue is the endothelium? Why would that make sense, particularly in a capillary?

_____

_____

_____

_____

Blood Vessel Identification

Activity Instructions

On the torso model, identify the structures listed in the left-hand column of the table below. As you identify each structure, write down the corresponding number in the right-hand column. Note: Many blood vessels are paired, meaning that there is a right vessel and a left vessel.

Table 18.2

Structure	Corresponding Number on Model
Ascending aorta	
Aortic arch	
Thoracic aorta	
Abdominal aorta	
Celiac trunk	
Superior mesenteric artery	
Inferior mesenteric artery	
Renal artery	
Common iliac artery	
External iliac artery	
Internal iliac artery	
Brachiocephalic trunk	
Subclavian artery	
Common carotid artery	
External carotid artery	
Internal carotid artery	

Table 18.2 (continued)

Structure	Corresponding Number on Model
Superior vena cava	
External jugular vein	
Internal jugular vein	
Brachiocephalic vein	
Subclavian vein	
Inferior vena cava	
Hepatic portal vein	
Hepatic vein	
Renal vein	
Common iliac vein	
External iliac vein	
Internal iliac vein	

Activity Questions

1. Name the three branches that come off the aortic arch.

_____

2. Most arteries and veins in a particular location share the same name; however, there are a few exceptions. Name the vessels you observed today that represent the exceptions.

_____

3. Use the models and Plate 11.03 in the textbook to describe blood flow through the hepatic portal system.

_____

_____

_____

_____

_____

Modeling of the Abdominal Aorta

You will use a Styrofoam rod and pipe cleaners to represent the abdominal aorta and its branches.

Activity Instructions

1. Obtain a sturdy, thick cylinder (rod) of Styrofoam. This represents the **abdominal aorta.** Insert an **orange** pipe cleaner into the superior portion of the cylinder.

2. Tie a **green** pipe cleaner around the left side of the orange pipe cleaner. Tie a **purple** pipe cleaner on the right side of the orange pipe cleaner. Tie a **pink** pipe cleaner around the orange pipe cleaner between the green and purple pipe cleaners.

3. Insert a **yellow** pipe cleaner an inch below the orange pipe cleaner and insert a **blue** pipe cleaner several inches inferior to the yellow pipe cleaner.

4. Insert two white pipe cleaners slightly below the yellow pipe cleaner on both sides of the Styrofoam rod.

Activity Questions

1. What abdominal aortic branch does the orange pipe cleaner represent?

_____

2. What vessel does the green pipe cleaner represent?

_____

3. What vessel does the purple pipe cleaner represent?

_____

4. What vessel does the pink pipe cleaner represent?

_____

5. What abdominal aortic branch does the yellow pipe cleaner represent?

_____

6. What abdominal aortic branch does the blue pipe cleaner represent?

_____

7. What vessels do the white pipe cleaners represent?

_____

Activity 18-6

Blood Vessel Mapping

Activity Instructions

Refer to Figures 11.22 and 11.23 and Plates 11.01, 11.02, 11.04 and 11.05 in your textbook.

1. Use your body outline from the bone mapping activity (Activity 11-2). If you did not do that activity, draw an outline of a body on a large piece of butcher paper and sketch in the clavicle, humerus, radius, ulna, femur, tibia, and fibula.

2. Work in groups of three. Use the anterior bone map. Even though you are working in groups of three, you need only one bone marking drawing.

3. Choose one group member to draw a heart in the correct location. It does not have to be completely anatomically correct. Just be sure to have the great vessels extending from the base.

4. Divide the tasks as follows:
   - Person 1: draw in the anterior arteries listed below in pencil first and then trace over the vessels with a **red** marker on the **right** of the anterior bone map.
   - Person 2: draw in the superficial veins listed below using a pencil first and then trace over the vessels with a **purple** marker on the **left** of the anterior bone map. This is the shortest list, so this person should also help persons 1 and 3 with their blood vessel drawings.
   - Person 3: draw in the deep veins listed below with a pencil first and then trace over the pencil marks with a **blue** marker on the **left** of the anterior bone map.
   - Be sure to use a pencil for your initial drawings so that you can erase and redraw any mistakes.
   - Number each vessel as you go and write the number of the vessel next to its name in the list below.
   - Use dotted lines to show vessels behind bones.

5. Quiz each other on the name of the vessels, using the key that you created to check answers.

Note: The vessels are listed in the order that you should draw them.

Arteries to Include

___ Ascending aorta	___ Facial artery
___ Aortic arch	___ Temporal artery
___ Brachiocephalic trunk	___ Abdominal artery
___ Subclavian artery	___ Renal artery
___ Axillary artery	___ Common iliac artery
___ Brachial artery	___ Internal iliac artery
___ Radial artery	___ External iliac artery
___ Ulnar artery	___ Deep femoral artery
___ Palmar arches	___ Femoral artery
___ Digital artery	___ Popliteal artery
___ Common carotid	___ Posterior tibial artery
___ Internal carotid artery	___ Anterior tibial artery
___ External carotid artery	___ Dorsalis pedis artery

Deep Veins to Include

___ Superior vena cava	___ Inferior vena cava
___ Subclavian vein	___ Renal vein
___ Brachiocephalic vein	___ Common iliac vein
___ Internal jugular vein	___ Internal iliac vein
___ External jugular vein	___ External iliac vein
___ Facial vein	___ Deep femoral vein
___ Temporal vein	___ Femoral vein
___ Brachial vein	___ Popliteal vein
___ Radial vein	___ Anterior tibial vein
___ Ulnar vein	___ Posterior tibial vein

Superficial Veins to Include

___ Cephalic vein
___ Basalic vein
___ Median cubital vein
___ Digital vein
___ Great saphenous vein
___ Small saphenous vein
___ Dorsal venous arch

Post-Lab Assessment

1. Which ventricle can generate a more forceful contraction?

   _____

2. Which great vessel is located most anteriorly on the heart?

   _____

3. How many brachiocephalic arteries are there? How many brachiocephalic veins are there? Explain the difference.

   _____

   _____

   _____

4. Name the vessel that receives the nutrient-rich blood from the digestive system organs and that enters the liver.

   _____

5. Trace the flow of blood from the left ventricle to the left kidney and back to the left ventricle

   _____

   _____

   _____

6. Trace the flow of blood from the left ventricle to the right fingers (take the medial pathway down the forearm) and back to the right atrium. Take the superficial, medial venous pathway up the arm.

   _____

   _____

7. Knowing what you know about blood flow through the heart and lungs, why does weakness of the heart muscle cause fluid backup (retention) in the lungs?

   _____

   _____

19

Cardiovascular Physiology

Textbook Correlation: Chapter 11—The Cardiovascular System

Details

Activities	Activity Objectives	Required Materials	Estimated Time
19-1: Electrocardiogram	Administer and interpret an electrocardiogram; relate events in the cardiac conduction system and the cardiac cycle to the peaks seen on the ECG	● Computer ● ECG sensor ● USB link ● Alcohol wipes ● 3 electrode patches	30 min
19-2: Heart Sounds	Identify heart sounds and relate the sounds to the closing of valves	● Alcohol wipes ● Stethoscope	10 min
19-3: Obtain a Blood Pressure Reading	Demonstrate the ability to take a blood pressure reading	● Alcohol wipes ● Stethoscope ● Sphygmomanometer	5–10 min
19-4: Effect of Activity Levels on Blood Pressure	Determine how increasing activity levels affect blood pressure; describe factors related to blood pressure	● Alcohol wipes ● Stethoscope ● Sphygmomanometer	30 min

Because of the nature of the activities performed in this lab, students should wear comfortable clothing and shoes that are comfortable to run in.

Overview

While watching a medical drama that shows a machine recording a patient's heart activity, have you ever wondered what the blips on the screen mean? The blips represent an electric recording of the heart, called an ECG (electrocardiogram). Electrocardiography is a convenient method for evaluating the functioning of the heart. Today you will perform this and other activities to evaluate the functioning of your own (or your lab partner's) cardiovascular system. So lace up your sneakers and let's get started!

Need to Know

- **Cardiac conduction system**
  - Series of specialized cardiac muscle cells specialized for impulse conduction
    - ○ **Sinoatrial (SA) node:** located in the wall of the right atrium
      - ■ First to fire the action potential and sends it to the atrioventricular node
    - ○ **Atrioventricular (AV) node:** located within the interatrial septum
      - ■ Delays impulse conduction; allows atria to contract before ventricles begin to contract
      - ■ Sends impulse to the atrioventricular bundle
    - ○ **Atrioventricular bundle:** carries the signal to the interventricular septum
      - ■ The only electrical connection between the atria and ventricles
    - ○ **Bundle branches:** extend from the interventricular septum to the apex; do not stimulate ventricular contraction
    - ○ **Purkinje fibers:** extend from the apex through the myocardium of the ventricle; stimulates myocardial contraction cells, beginning at the apex

- **ECG:** registers the electrical changes in many heart muscle cells over the course of each heart beat
  - Also known as an **EKG** (from the German *Elektrokardiogramm*).
  - **P wave:** atrial depolarization.
  - **QRS wave:** ventricular depolarization and atrial repolarization.
  - **T wave:** ventricular repolarization.
  - The time interval between the P wave and the QRS wave represents the atrial action potential.
    - ○ Provides a rough estimate of atrial contraction duration
  - The time interval between the QRS complex and the T wave represents the ventricular action potential.
    - ○ Provides a rough estimate of ventricular contraction duration

- **Heart sounds:**
  - **S1:** Louder of the two sounds (the "lub" sound)
    - ○ Due to the closing of the atrioventricular valves
  - **S2:** Softer of the two sounds ("dub")
    - ○ Due to the closing of the semilunar valves

- **Blood pressure:**
  - Pressure in the systemic arteries is measured to determine the risk of cardiovascular disease
  - Arterial blood pressure reflects:
    - Arterial compliance (stretchiness); only varies with disease
    - Arterial blood volume, which increases if
      - More blood enters the arteries (increased cardiac output); reflects increased stroke volume and/or increased heart rate. The sympathetic nervous system increases both heart rate and stroke volume.
      - Less blood leaves the arteries; results from vasoconstriction (narrowing) in the arterioles. The sympathetic nervous system stimulates vasoconstriction.
  - Arterial blood pressure varies over the cardiac cycle.
    - **Systolic pressure:** the large surge in pressure resulting from left ventricular contraction
    - **Diastolic pressure:** lower pressure due to the recoiling of the artery as the blood moves forward
    - **Pulse pressure:** the difference between systolic and diastolic pressure
    - **Sphygmomanometer:** instrument with an inflatable cuff and pressure gauge that measures arterial blood pressure

Pre-Lab Activity

Students should complete this activity before completing the lab activities that follow.

1. Label the following picture of the cardiac conduction system using the following terms (add your own leader lines):
   - Atrioventricular branches
   - Atrioventricular node
   - Bundle branches
   - Purkinje fibers
   - Sinoatrial node

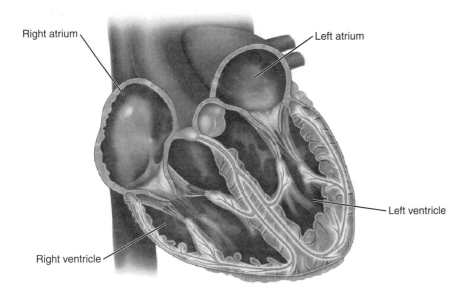

2. Label the waves and segments in the ECG diagram below:
   - P wave
   - QRS wave
   - T wave
   - P-Q segment
   - Q-T segment

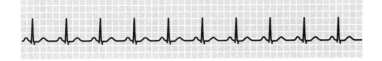

Electrocardiogram (ECG)

Activity Instructions

Work in groups of two to four and obtain ECG readings for one or all members of the group. If your institution uses sensors other than the PASCO sensors, your instructor will provide you with a different set of instructions.

1. Turn on the computer and plug the USB link into the USB port on the computer.

2. Plug the ECG sensor into the USB link.

3. Click on the "Data Studio" icon on the desktop and then click the "Open Activity" folder. Click the "EKG" lab.

4. Choose a subject. The subject must remove all jewelry and metal from the body (including piercings).

5. Use the alcohol wipes to sanitize the right wrist, right forearm (just below the elbow), and left forearm (just below the elbow).

6. Place the electrode patches on the subject in the areas mentioned above.

7. Locate the alligator clips on the ECG sensor and attach the clips to the patches in the following order:
   a. Black lead (ground): right wrist
   b. Green lead (negative): right forearm
   c. Red lead (positive): left forearm

8. Look at the LED light on the ECG sensor. It should be flashing on and off in rhythm with the heartbeat. The flashing light indicates that the sensor is ready to collect data.

9. Instruct the subject to sit still and refrain from talking, laughing, nervous movements, and so on.

10. When the subject is ready, click the "Start" button on the main tool bar. You will see waves forming on the graph over the next 14 seconds (Data Studio automatically records the data).

11. Send the ECG results to the printer and collect the printout. Do not exit from Data Studio yet.

12. Calculate the subject's heart rate by using the printout. Count the number of "peaks" (top of the QRS wave) that occur during a 6-second interval (number of beats in 6 seconds). Multiply the number obtained by 10 for the beats per minute. Record in the table below.

13. Check the accuracy of your calculation by clicking the "Restore Down" button on the upper right corner of your reading (Graph 2) (not the white icon on the Data Studio window). If you clicked on the correct button, you should see a reading of the subject's heart rate. Record it in Table 19.1.

14. If you have time to perform an ECG on other group members, click the "Maximize" button in the upper right corner of the "Graph 2" window and a new graph should appear.

15. Repeat steps 4 through 13 with the next subject. Since alcohol wipes are used on the skin, it is acceptable to reuse the same electrode patches.

16. When your group is finished, ask your instructor if you should save your data on the hard drive or quit the program without saving your data.

Table 19.1 Heart Rate Data	
Calculated Heart Rate	**Computer-Derived Heart Rate**

Activity Questions

1. Label the P wave, QRS complex, and T wave on the ECG printout and attach it to your lab report.

2. Determine the P-Q segment (beginning of P wave to beginning of the drop in the Q wave) by counting the number of boxes between the two points. Record the number on the lines below and explain what this number represents.

_____

_____

3. Determine the Q-T segment (beginning of QRS complex to the end of the T wave) by counting the number of boxes between the two points. Record the number on the lines below and explain what this number represents.

_____

_____

4. Fill in Table 19.2. (The first line is completed as an example.)

Table 19.2 The Electrocardiograph	Electrical Events in the Cardiac Muscle	Events in the Cardiac Cycle
P wave	Atria are depolarizing	Atrial systole (contraction begins)
QRS complex		
T wave		

Heart Sounds

In this activity you will perform a clinical technique called **auscultation,** which uses a stethoscope to listen to sounds in the thoracic cavity. By placing the stethoscope in specific locations, you will hear the sounds of heart valves closing. It is important to note that sounds travel through the chest, and the stethoscope placements do not correspond to the location of the actual valves.

Activity Instructions

1. If you have Internet access, use this URL to listen to the sounds of the heart: http://depts.washington.edu/physdx/heart/demo.html. If the link does not work, do a search for "heart sounds examples."

2. Choose a subject and instruct him or her to sit still; obtain alcohol wipes and a stethoscope.

3. Use the alcohol wipes to clean the stethoscope ear buds and diaphragm.

4. Put the ear buds in your ears. Place the diaphragm of the stethoscope over the subject's second intercostal space, at the right upper sternal border. Listen for the lub (S1)-dub (S2) sounds. Answer the following two activity questions.

Activity Questions

1. Which sound is louder: S1 or S2?

_____

2. Which group of valves is closing during the louder sound?

_____

Obtain a Blood Pressure Reading

This activity uses auscultation to determine blood pressure. See Figure 11.20 in your textbook to help you perform this activity and interpret your results. If your institution uses a different technique, your instructor will provide you with a different protocol to obtain your readings. Be sure that the chosen subject can perform vigorous exercise.

Activity Instructions

It is important to master this skill so that you can complete the next lab activity.

1. Work in groups of two to four students.

2. Choose the subject and instruct him or her to find a quiet place to lie down while you and the rest of your group prep the subject for the blood pressure reading. Instruct the subject to remain silent.

3. Use the alcohol wipes to clean the ear buds and the diaphragm of the stethoscope and put the ear buds in your ears.

4. Obtain the subject's pulse (heart rate) by placing your index and middle fingers on the radial pulse pressure point. Do not use your thumb. Count the number of beats in one minute. Record in Table 19.3.

5. Wrap the sphygmomanometer around the subject's left arm in the brachial region (approximately 1 in. above the antecubital area).

6. Locate the subject's pulse in the antecubital area (the brachial artery) with the diaphragm of the stethoscope.

Safety Alert: The following steps must be completed within 1 minute. If not completed within that time, release the pressure in the sphygmomanometer and start over. **It is very important to read the following instructions before proceeding.**

7. Occlude the brachial artery by pumping up the cuff to 160 to 200 mm Hg. The cuff is inflated to a high pressure to cut off blood flow through the brachial artery. At this point, you should not hear anything because blood is not flowing through the artery.

8. Gradually decrease the pressure in the cuff while listening for the first sound (Korotkoff sound). This sound results from turbulent blood flow through the artery. It is first heard when cuff pressure falls just below systolic pressure.
   - The number on the pressure gauge at which this sound is heard is the systolic pressure. Record the number in the table below.

9. Continue releasing the pressure in the cuff gradually until the sound disappears; this is due to the pressure in the cuff falling below diastolic pressure. Blood now flows freely through the artery.
   ● The number on the pressure gauge at which sounds disappear is the diastolic pressure. Write down this value in the diastolic pressure column.

10. Tell the subject to remain supine until you start the next activity.

11. Calculate pulse pressure, which is the difference between systolic pressure and diastolic pressure ($P_{systole} - P_{diastole}$).

Table 19.3 Blood Pressure Results at Rest			
Heart Rate (beats per minute)	Systolic Pressure (mm Hg)	Diastolic Pressure (mm Hg)	Pulse Pressure (mm Hg)

Activity Questions

1. What is considered to be the normal blood pressure value? Was the subject's blood pressure within the normal range? The normal range for blood pressure is from 130/85 to 110/75.

   _____

   _____

2. If you obtained a blood pressure reading of 160/95 mm Hg, what are some factors that could result in the elevated number? List at least four.

   _____

   _____

   _____

   _____

3. **Critical Thinking:** Why is an artery used instead of a vein in obtaining a blood pressure reading?

   _____

   _____

   _____

   _____

   _____

Effect of Activity Levels on Blood Pressure

Students will take blood pressure readings from a subject immediately after the subject performs four different activities that increase in intensity. The final (fifth) reading is to determine blood pressure 10 minutes after intense exercise.

Activity Instructions

Use the same subject for this activity as you did for Activity 19-3.

1. In Table 19.4, record the heart rate and blood pressure reading from Activity 19-3 in the "Lying Down" row.

2. Instruct the subject to sit quietly upright for 5 minutes.

3. Take the subject's heart rate and blood pressure (following the technique explained in the previous activity) and record them in the table below.

4. Instruct the subject to walk briskly around the lab or in the hallway for 5 minutes. The subject should walk as fast as he or she would if running late for class. Obtain the subject's heart rate and blood pressure and record them in the table below.

5. Instruct the subject to exercise vigorously for 5 minutes, perhaps by running or climbing stairs. Measure the heart rate and blood pressure after the 5 minutes and record them in the table below.

6. Instruct the subject to rest for 10 minutes and take the heart rate and blood pressure again. Record the readings in the table.

7. Calculate the pulse pressure for each activity. The pulse pressure is the difference between systolic pressure and diastolic pressure.

Table 19.4 Blood Pressure Data with Increasing Activity				
Activity	**Heart Rate (beats per minute)**	**Systole (mm Hg)**	**Diastole (mm Hg)**	**Pulse Pressure**
Lying down				
Sitting up				
Walking briskly				
Running				
Recovery				

Activity Questions

1. Which activity was the subject performing when blood pressure was lowest? Highest? Are the data consistent with the expected outcome?

   _____

   _____

2. Will arterioles in working skeletal muscles dilate or constrict during increased activity? Why?

   _____

   _____

   _____

   _____

3. How do increased activity levels affect venous return? Explain your answer.

   _____

   _____

   _____

4. Which specific division of the nervous system is responsible for the response seen with increasing activity levels?

   _____

5. **Critical Thinking:** During which activity was pulse pressure the greatest? Why do you think so? Which number (systolic or diastolic) changed the most?

   _____

   _____

   _____

   _____

   _____

   _____

6. **Critical Thinking:** How did the heart rate change with increasing activity levels? How did this change in heart rate alter filling time and preload?

_____

_____

_____

_____

_____

_____

Post-Lab Assessment

1. Explain why the value for systolic blood pressure is higher than the value for diastolic blood pressure.

_____

_____

_____

_____

2. Make a flowchart that shows the sequence in which electrical impulses travel through the cardiac conduction system.

_____

_____

_____

3. Relate the events that occur during the cardiac cycle to the sounds heard through the stethoscope.

_____

_____

_____

_____

4. **Critical Thinking:** What does it mean when a person gets a pacemaker? Name the structure that is not working properly and explain why that structure is important.

_____

_____

_____

_____

5. **Critical Thinking:** Look at the ECG below and compare it with the ECG in the pre-lab activity. How is it different? What might this indicate?

_____

_____

_____

_____

Fill in the following statements using the terms listed below. Not all of the terms will be used.

Blood pressure
Contractility
Diastole
ECG
Heart rate
Parasympathetic division
Preload
Pulse pressure
QRS complex
Skeletal muscle pump
Sympathetic division
Systole

6. Instrument that detects the electrical currents produced by the heart: _____

7. Relaxation of the heart chambers: _____

8. Number of times the heart beats per minute: _____

9. The force the blood exerts against the vessel wall: _____

10. The difference between the systolic pressure and the diastolic pressure: _____

11. The name of the mechanism whereby the contraction of skeletal muscle promotes blood returning to the heart: _____

12. Contraction of heart chambers; most detectable in the left ventricle: _____

13. The maximum amount of blood that the ventricles contain prior to contraction: _____

14. The large surge on an ECG reading that represents the beginning of ventricular depolarization: _____

15. The division of the nervous system that increases heart rate and contractility: _____

20

Lymphatic System Anatomy

Textbook Correlation: Chapter 12—Immunity and the Lymphatic System

Details

Activities	Activity Objectives	Required Materials	Estimated Time
20-1: Lymphatic System: Gross Anatomy	Discribe the gross anatomy of the lymphatic organs	● Head model ● Torso model	15 min
20-2: Lymphatic System: Microscopic Anatomy	Discribe the microscopic anatomy of the lymphatic organs	● Microscope ● Thymus slide ● Spleen slide ● Lymph node slide	25 min
20-3: Lymphatic Vessel Tracing	Trace the flow of lymph through lymphatic vessels and lymph nodes; identify the veins that receive the lymph	● Blood vessel map (activity 18-5) ● Pencil ● Markers (light green, dark green, orange, blue, pink, purple, yellow, black)	35 min
20-4: Lymph Formation Modeling	Describe the formation of lymph, relating it to the pressures operating in a blood capillary	● Markers (black, red, dark blue, light blue, purple, green, orange)	30 min

Overview

It was once thought that many of the lymphatic organs were not necessary and could be removed without consequence. For example, a few decades ago, it was routine for 8- to 10-year-old children to undergo a tonsillectomy, or removal of the tonsils. It was believed that the tonsils had no function and acted as "microbe incubators." We now understand that tonsils are the site of initial encounters between leukocytes and air- and foodborne pathogens. Tonsils are now removed only if they become inflamed and impede breathing and swallowing.

The appendix is another example. Until recently, it was thought to be a *vestigial organ*; that is, an organ whose function had lost importance as humans evolved. We now recognize the appendix as an important reservoir of protective bacteria that can restore our gut flora in the case of severe diarrhea. Diarrhea flushes out the healthy gut bacteria, which ferment food products and synthesize (activate) vitamin K. The appendix stores "reserve" bacteria that can quickly replace the lost bacteria and restore homeostasis.

The lymphatic and immune systems are closely linked. The lymphatic system contains organs and immune cells, whereas the immune system is a diverse group of cells and chemicals that accomplish a common function. (Note that the lymphatic system also has functions unrelated to immunity, such as fluid balance and the absorption of fat-soluble vitamins). Today's lab focuses on the gross and microscopic anatomy of the lymphatic system and the formation and flow of lymph.

Need to Know

- **Lymphatic system organs:**
  - **Spleen:** located in the abdominal cavity, superior to the left adrenal gland and posterior to the stomach
    - ○ **Red pulp:** contains large venous sinuses separated by cords of tissue; erythrocytes, lymphocytes, and macrophages are suspended on the cords.
    - ○ **White pulp:** contains collections of lymphocytes and macrophages that surround the splenic arteries.
  - **Thymus:** located posterior to the sternum, covering the distal portion of the trachea and base of the heart.
    - ○ Houses and matures T lymphocytes
    - ○ Grows until puberty; subsequently shrinks and is eventually replaced by adipose tissue
    - ○ Anatomy:
      - ■ **Lobules:** divisions, or sections, of the thymus
      - ■ **Cortex:** superficial regions of the organ
      - ■ **Medulla:** deeper region containing tightly packed cells
  - **Lymph nodes:** clusters of small nodules located in the network of lymphatic vessels (see below)
    - ○ **Afferent vessels:** carry lymph into lymph node
    - ○ **Capsule:** fibrous tissue that connects the lymph node to the surrounding structures
    - ○ **Cortex:** outer portion of the node (beneath the capsule) that contains:
      - ■ **Follicles:** clusters of lymphocytes; **germinal centers** are darker-staining sections of the follicles that contain multiplying B lymphocytes
    - ○ **Medulla:** deep region of the lymph node
      - ■ **Medullary cords:** contain lymphocytes and macrophages suspended on reticular fibers (cords)
      - ■ **Medullary sinuses:** spaces between the cords through which the lymph flows

○ **Efferent vessels:** transport lymph out of the lymph node
  ■ Fewer efferent vessels than afferent vessels means that lymph flow slows through the node, permitting adequate processing time

● **Mucosa-Associated Lymphoid Tissue (MALT):**
  ● Collection (aggregates) of lymphoid tissue strategically located at major entry points for pathogens (respiratory and gastrointestinal tracts)
  ● **Tonsils:** line the oral cavity and pharynx
    ○ **Palatine tonsils:** located on either side of the posterior portion of the oral cavity
      ■ Large and easy to see, particularly in tonsillitis (inflammation of the tonsils); attack food-borne pathogens
    ○ **Pharyngeal tonsil:** located on the posterior wall of the nasopharynx
      ■ Hidden; attacks airborne pathogens
  ● **Appendix:** small, wormlike structure that hangs off the large intestine
    ○ Contains a collection of lymphoid tissue and houses symbiotic (helpful) bacteria
  ● **Peyer's patches:** found in the wall of the small intestine
    ○ Number of patches increases as the small intestine gets closer to the large intestine and appendix

● **Lymph formation:** Lymph vessels carry **lymph:** a watery fluid similar to plasma but with fewer proteins
  ● Lymph forms in tissues from filtered capillary blood
    ○ **Hydrostatic pressure:** high on the arteriole side of the capillary
      ■ Pressure in capillary is higher than pressure in surrounding interstitial fluid (ISF)
      ■ Pushes water and small solutes into the ISF
    ○ **Osmotic pressure:** high on the venule side of the capillary
      ■ Low water concentration and high albumin (protein) concentration in the capillary
      ■ Draws (reabsorbs) some (but not all) of the filtered water back into the capillary
  ● Filtered fluid that is not reabsorbed forms lymph

● **Lymph transport:**
  ● **Lymphatic capillaries:** blunt-ended capillaries that begin in tissues
    ○ High pressure interstitial fluid pushes open flaps between the endothelial cells in the lymphatic capillaries.
    ○ Lymph enters lymphatic capillary until pressure in lymphatic capillary equals pressure in ISF.
  ● **Lymphatic vessels:** highly branched lymph transport vessels
    ○ Carry lymph under low pressure, in many cases against gravity
    ○ Contain valves:
      ■ Help to transport lymph in one direction, toward the heart
      ■ Skeletal muscle pump, as in veins, assists in lymph transport
  ● **Lymphatic ducts:** transport lymph from the lymphatic vessels to the veins
    ○ **Right lymphatic duct:** drains lymph coming from the right arm, right side of the chest, and right side of the head and neck
      ■ Feeds into the **right subclavian vein**
    ○ **Thoracic duct:** drains the rest (majority) of the body
      ■ Feeds into the **left subclavian vein**
  ● The lymph now becomes part of the venous blood.

Pre-Lab Activity

Students should complete this activity before completing the lab activities that follow.

1. What do you think is a function of the spleen, based on the types of cells it contains?

   _____

   _____

2. Label the accompanying figure with the following terms:
   - Capsule
   - Cortex
   - Lobule
   - Medulla
   - Red pulp
   - Sinus
   - Spleen
   - Splenic cord
   - Thymus
   - White pulp

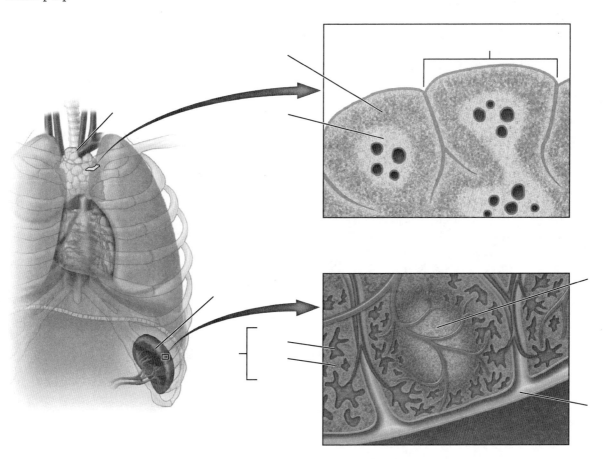

3. Label the accompanying figure with the following terms:
    - Axillary node
    - Cervical node
    - Inguinal node
    - Lymphatic vessels
    - Submandibular node
    - Thoracic duct

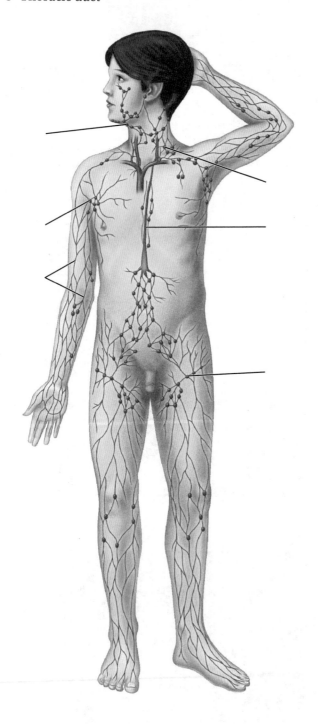

Lymphatic Organ Gross Anatomy

Activity Instructions

On the torso and head models, identify the organs listed in the left-hand column of Table 20-1 and write the corresponding number in the right-hand column of the table. Refer to Figures 12-7 and 12-8 in your textbook.

Table 20.1 Lymphatic Organs and Structures	
Organ/MALT	**Corresponding Number on Model**
Appendix	
Spleen	
Palatine tonsil	
Pharyngeal tonsil	

Activity Questions

1. Describe the specific location of the spleen.

   _____

   _____

2. The appendix "hangs" off of (or is suspended by) one organ. Name this organ.

   _____

3. Name the tonsil that is closest to incoming air from the nasal cavity.

   _____

4. Name the group of tonsils on the lateral sides of the oropharynx (the entrance of the nasal cavity into the throat). What is their function, based on the location?

   _____

   _____

Microscopic Lymphatic Anatomy

Activity Instructions

Identify the following microscopic organs and structures. Draw, label, and describe your findings. Refer to Figures 12-6 and 12-7 in your textbook.

1. Identify the following structures on the lymph node slide under both scanning and low powers. Draw, label, and describe your findings in the spaces provided.
   - Capsule
   - Cortex
     - Lymphoid follicles
       - ○ Germinal centers
   - Medulla
     - Medullary cords
     - Medullary sinuses

TM _____

Slide name _____

Description _____

_____

_____

_____

_____

TM _____

Slide name _____

Description _____

_____

_____

_____

2. Identify the following structures on the thymus slide under both scanning and low powers. Draw, label, and describe your findings in the spaces provided.
   ● Lobule
   ● Cortex
   ● Medulla

TM _____

Slide name _____

Description _____

_____

_____

_____

_____

TM _____

Slide name _____

Description _____

_____

_____

_____

_____

3. Identify the following structures on the spleen slide under low power. Draw, label, and describe your findings in the spaces provided.
   ● Red pulp
   ● White pulp

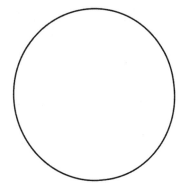

TM _____

Slide name _____

Description _____

_____

_____

_____

4. Identify the following structure on the small intestine slide under low power. Draw, label, and describe your findings in the space provided.
   - Peyer's patches

TM _____

Slide name _____

Description _____

_____

_____

_____

_____

Activity Questions

1. Name the lymphocyte found in the germinal centers of the lymph nodes.

_____

2. Name the structure in the medulla of the lymph nodes that contains the leukocytes.

_____

3. Name the type of fiber found in the medulla of the lymph node.

_____

4. Name the lymphocyte that matures in the thymus.

_____

5. Is the thymus easily visible in the elderly?

_____

6. Compare the blood cell components of the white pulp and red pulp of the spleen.

_____

_____

_____

Lymphatic Vessel Tracing

Activity Instructions

Working in pairs, add the lymphatic vessels, nodes, and ducts to your blood-tracing map from Activity 18-5. You may prefer to make a new body outline for this activity, which will later be used in future labs. Refer to Figures 12-5 and 12-6 in the textbook.

1. Use a pencil to draw in a series of lymphatic vessels throughout the legs, arms, abdomen, neck, and face.

2. Draw the right lymphatic duct and the thoracic duct, ensuring that each duct is emptying into the correct vein. If you are using a new body tracing, add in the brachiocephalic veins and the inferior vena cava.

3. Use your pencil to draw clusters of circles to represent the lymph nodes along the lymphatic vessels. Be sure to draw large clusters in the inguinal, axillary, and cervical regions.

4. Once you are satisfied with your lymphatic vessels, ducts, and nodes, trace over the pencil marks. Use a **light green** marker to represent lymphatic vessels that merge into the right lymphatic duct. Use a **dark green** marker to represent lymphatic vessels that merge into the thoracic duct.

5. To the right of your body tracing, draw an enlarged lymph node in pencil. Refer to Figure 12-6 in your textbook and your drawing of the lymph node in the previous activity. Include the afferent and efferent vessels with valves.

6. Color the germinal centers **purple** and the surrounding follicles **pink.**

7. Color the medullary cords **blue.**

8. Color the afferent vessels **orange** and the efferent vessels **yellow.**

9. Draw an arrow in **black** showing the direction that lymph takes through the lymph node.

Activity Questions

1. Which vein receives lymph from the right lymphatic duct?

_____

2. Which vein receives lymph from the thoracic duct?

_____

3. Which duct receives lymph from the majority of the body?

_____

4. Lymphatic vessels have valves. What other vessels contain valves?

_____

5. Why do you think that lymphatic vessels have valves? List two reasons.

_____

_____

6. Name the organ that all lymphatic vessels travel toward.

_____

7. **Critical Thinking:** The function of the lymph node is to process the lymph by screening out pathogens and tumor cells. There are more afferent vessels than efferent vessels. Why do you think that is true?

_____

_____

_____

_____

_____

Activity 20-4

Lymph Formation

Activity Instructions

Refer to Figures 11-15 and 12-4 in your textbook.

1. Draw a capillary in **black** in the space below and label the left side of the capillary "A" (for arteriole end) in **red**. Label the right side of the capillary "V" (for venule end) in **dark blue**. Label the space surrounding the capillary "ISF" (for interstitial fluid).

2. Answer activity question 1 and write ↑HP (for high hydrostatic pressure) in the capillary on the side that has the higher hydrostatic pressure.

3. Answer activity question 2.

4. Illustrate your answer to question 2 by drawing a **light-blue** arrow illustrating fluid movement.

5. Answer question 3 and write ↑OP (for osmotic pressure) in the capillary on the side that has the higher osmotic pressure.

6. Illustrate your answer to question 3 by drawing a **purple** arrow illustrating fluid movement.

7. Answer question 4.

8. Use a **green** marker to draw a lymphatic capillary in the interstitial fluid. Be sure to draw some spaces in between the endothelial cells.

9. Answer question 5.

10. Illustrate your answer to question 5 by drawing an **orange** arrow illustrating fluid movement.

Activity Questions

1. Which side of the capillary has a higher hydrostatic pressure: the side closer to the arteriole or the side closer to the venule? Why?

_____

_____

_____

_____

2. What occurs to the fluid in the capillary where the hydrostatic pressure is high?

3. Does the hydrostatic pressure increase or decrease in relation to the osmotic pressure on the venule side? Why? In which direction will the fluid move?

4. Does all fluid that was pushed into the interstitial fluid get reclaimed (absorbed) on the venule side?

5. What happens to fluid that is not reclaimed by the blood capillary? Explain the path that it takes.

Post-Lab Assessment

1. **Critical Thinking:** Many breast cancer patients have lymph nodes and lymphatic vessels removed from the axillary region and many uterine cancer patients have lymph nodes removed from the inguinal region. Why do you think that lymph nodes are removed from those specific locations?

_____

_____

_____

_____

2. **Critical Thinking:** Some breast cancer and uterine cancer survivors will suffer from **lymphedema,** which is massive swelling that can becaused by the removal of lymphatic vessels. Lymphedema is typically seen in the arm in breast cancer survivors or thigh in uterine cancer survivors. Why do you think lymphedema occurs?

_____

_____

_____

_____

3. **Critical Thinking:** Most nutrients have been absorbed by the time the unabsorbed food residue enters the large intestine. The large intestine contains a population of symbiotic bacteria that remain in the large intestine. As the small intestine gets closer to the large intestine, the number of Peyer's patches increases. Why do you think that makes sense?

_____

_____

_____

_____

21

Respiratory System Anatomy

Textbook Correlation: Chapter 13—The Respiratory System

Details

Activities	Activity Objectives	Required Materials	Estimated Time
21-1: Upper Respiratory System Anatomy	Identify the cavities and structures of the upper respiratory tract	● Midsagittal head model ● Frontal head model	20 min
21-2: Lower Respiratory System Anatomy	Identify the organs and structures of the lower respiratory tract	● Midsagittal head model ● Larynx model ● Lung model	20 min
21-3: Respiratory System: Microscopic Anatomy	Describe the microscopic anatomy of the respiratory organs and structures	● Microscopic lung anatomy model ● Microscope ● Lung slide ● Lung carcinoma slide ● Trachea slide	20 min
21-4: Body Mapping	Draw and identify the organs of the respiratory system	● Large butcher paper ● Pencil ● Markers	35 min

Overview

Strep throat, sinus infection, laryngitis, bronchitis, rhinitis, influenza—these are all common infections of the respiratory tract. But what, exactly, are the structures of the respiratory system that are affected by each of these illnesses? Today's lab focuses on the anatomical structures of the respiratory system; the next lab will focus on the physiology of the respiratory system.

Need to Know

Conducting zone: conducts air but does not participate in gas exchange

- With the exception of the oropharynx, the conducting zone is lined by **respiratory epithelium**
  - Composed of **ciliated pseudostratified columnar epithelium**
  - **Goblet cells:** interspersed between ciliated cells
  - Mucus secreted by the goblet cells traps inhaled dust particles and pathogens, and the cilia sweep the mucus toward the nasal or oral cavity.

- **Nasal cavity:** space through which air enters the body via the **nostrils** (openings into the nasal cavity)
  - Formed by:
    - **Palate:** separates the nasal cavity from the oral cavity
      - Hard palate: maxillae and palatine bones
      - Soft palate: muscle; extends posteriorly and inferiorly as the **uvula**
    - **Nasal septum:** separates the right and left nasal cavities
    - **Nasal conchae:** three shelflike structures located on the lateral walls of each cavity
  - **Paranasal sinuses:** hollow cavities that form a ring around the nasal cavity—named for the bones in which they are located
    - **Sphenoid sinus**
    - **Maxillary sinus**
    - **Frontal sinus**
    - **Ethmoid air cells**

- **Pharynx:**
  - **Nasopharynx:** superior portion
    - Posterior to the nasal cavity
    - Contains the **pharyngeal tonsil**
  - **Oropharynx:** middle portion
    - Extends from the uvula to the tongue, posterior to the oral cavity
    - Lined by stratified squamous epithelium
    - Contains the **palatine tonsils** and the **lingual tonsil**
  - **Laryngopharynx:** inferior portion
    - Extends to the larynx
    - Wall is continuous with the oropharynx

- **Larynx:** commonly known as the voice box; anterior to the laryngopharynx
  - **Epiglottis:** flap of elastic cartilage that covers the larynx during swallowing
  - **Thyroid cartilage:** hyaline cartilage that forms the majority of the V-shaped larynx
    - Enlarges in males, forming the "Adam's apple"
  - **Cricoid cartilage:** small ring of hyaline cartilage inferior to the thyroid cartilage

- **Trachea:** commonly known as the windpipe; extends inferiorly from the larynx
  - Contains 16 to 20 C-shaped rings of hyaline cartilage

- **Bronchial tree:** conducts air from the trachea to the air sacs of the lungs
  - **Mainstem (primary) bronchi:** branch directly from the trachea
    - ○ Right mainstem bronchus enters the right lung; left mainstem bronchus enters the left lung
  - **Lobar (secondary) bronchi:** two to three branches off of each mainstem bronchus
  - **Segmental (tertiary) bronchi:** branches of each lobar bronchus
  - **Bronchioles:** very small air-conducting tubes (diameter >1 mm)
  - **Terminal bronchioles:** smallest tubes that bring air toward the air sacs

Respiratory zone: gas-exchange area of the lungs

- **Respiratory bronchioles:** very small tubes that give rise to the air sacs

- **Alveoli:** small air sacs that allow for gas exchange between the lungs and the pulmonary capillaries

Lungs: large, light organs responsible for gas exchange with the external environment

- **Right lung:** larger of the two lungs; has three lobes:
  - **Superior lobe**
  - **Middle lobe:** a horizontal fissure separates the superior lobe from the middle lobe.
  - **Inferior lobe**

- **Left lung:** has only two lobes (no middle lobe)

- **Serous membranes:** surround the lungs
  - **Visceral pleura:** serous membrane layer in direct contact with the surface of the lung
  - **Parietal pleura:** serous membrane layer attached to the rib cage, diaphragm, and the fibrous pericardium
  - **Intrapleural space:** fluid-filled very narrow space between the two pleural membranes

Pre-Lab Activity

Students should complete this activity before completing the lab activities that follow.

Match the following structures with the correct categorization in the respiratory tract.

A. Lower respiratory tract

B. Upper respiratory tract

1. Mainstem bronchi: _____

2. Ethmoid air cells: _____

3. Frontal sinus: _____

4. Laryngopharynx: _____

5. Larynx: _____

6. Lungs: _____

7. Maxillary sinus: _____

8. Nasal cavity: _____

9. Nasopharynx: _____

10. Nose: _____

11. Oropharynx: _____

12. Trachea: _____

13. Identify the structures listed above on the diagrams below. Some terms may be used more than once. Include these terms as well:
- Cricoid cartilage
- Epiglottis
- Nasal conchae
- Hard palate
- Soft palate
- Thyroid cartilage

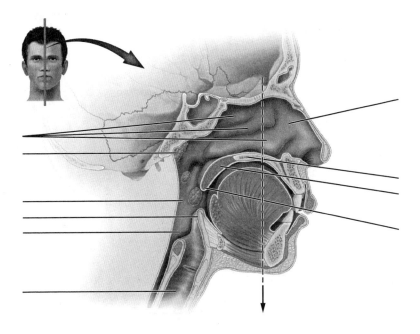

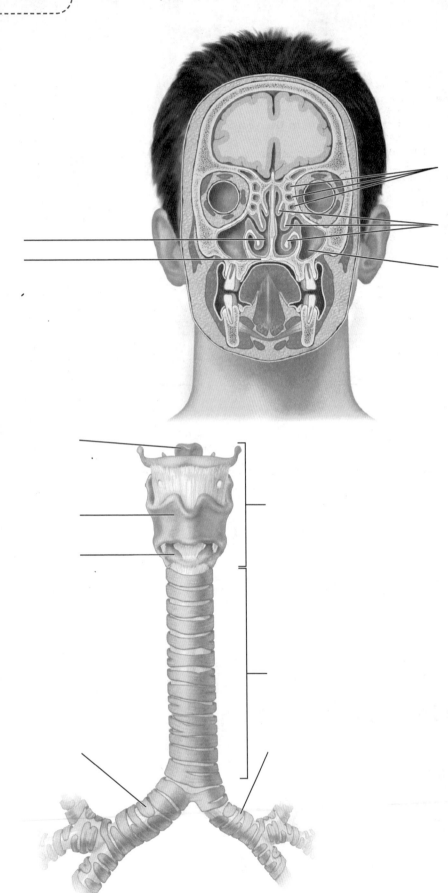

Upper Respiratory System Anatomy

Activity Instructions

On the midsagittal and frontal head models, identify the organs and structures listed in the left-hand column of Table 21.1. As you identify each structure, write down the corresponding number in the right-hand column. Name the model that you used to identify each organ or structure in the middle column. Refer to Figure 13-4 in the textbook.

Table 21.1 Upper Respiratory System Structures		
Structure	**Relevant Model (frontal or midsagittal)**	**Corresponding Number on Model**
External Nose		
Nasal bone		
Nasal cartilage		
Nostril		
Internal Nose (Nasal Cavity)		
Hard palate		
Soft palate		
Uvula		
Bony nasal septum		
Superior nasal concha		
Middle nasal concha		
Inferior nasal concha		

(continued)

Table 21.1 Upper Respiratory System Structures (continued)		
Structure	**Relevant Model (frontal or midsagittal)**	**Corresponding Number on Model**
Paranasal sinuses		
Frontal sinus		
Sphenoid sinus		
Maxillary sinus		
Ethmoid air cells		
Pharynx		
Nasopharynx		
Pharyngeal tonsil		
Oropharynx		
Palatine tonsils		
Laryngopharynx		

Activity Questions

1. Name the paranasal sinus located below the eye orbit.

_____

2. Name the lymphatic structures identified in the model.

_____

3. Name the specific region of the tube located inferior to the oropharynx.

_____

4. Name the holes through which air enters the nasal cavity.

_____

5. Name the two bones that form the nasal septum.

_____

Lower Respiratory System Anatomy

Activity Instructions

On the midsagittal head, larynx, and lower respiratory system models, identify the organs and structures listed in the left-hand column of Table 21.2. As you identify each structure, write down the corresponding number in the right-hand column. Name the model that you used to identify each organ or structure in the middle column. Refer to Figures 13-4, 13-5, 13-6, and 13-7 in your textbook.

Table 21.2 Lower Respiratory System Structures		
Structure	**Relevant Model**	**Corresponding Number on the Model**
Larynx		
Epiglottis		
Thyroid cartilage		
Cricoid cartilage		
Vestibular folds (false vocal cords)		
Vestibular cords (true vocal cords)		
Trachea		
Tracheal cartilage rings		
Trachealis muscle		
Mainstem (primary) bronchi (left and right)		
Lobar (secondary) bronchi		
Segmental (tertiary) bronchi		

(continued)

Table 21.2   Lower Respiratory System Structures (continued)

Structure	Relevant Model	Corresponding Number on the Model
Lungs (right and left)		
Superior lobe		
Middle lobe		
Inferior lobe		
Visceral pleura		
Diaphragm		

Activity Questions

1. How many lobar bronchi are there on the right side (in the right lung)? What about the left lung? Why is there a difference?

_____

_____

_____

2. Describe the difference in location between the thyroid cartilage and the cricoid cartilage.

_____

_____

_____

3. Name the organ system that includes the diaphragm. Why do you think that the diaphragm is discussed in this chapter?

_____

_____

_____

4. **Critical Thinking:** The laryngopharynx routes food and liquids down one tube and air down another tube. Which tube does air enter? Which tube does food and liquid enter? What structure in the larynx routes air, food, and liquid down the appropriate tube?

_____

_____

_____

Activity 21-3

Microscopic Anatomy

Activity Instructions

1. On the microscopic lung anatomy model, identify the structures listed in the left-hand column of Table 21.3. As you identify each structure, write down the corresponding number in the right-hand column. Refer to Figure 13-6 in the textbook.

Table 21.3

Structure	Corresponding Number on Model
Terminal bronchiole	
Respiratory bronchiole	
Alveolar duct	
Alveolus	

2. Identify the **alveolus** on the lung slide under high power. Draw, label, and describe your findings.

TM _____

Slide name _____

Description _____

_____

_____

_____

_____

3. Observe the lung carcinoma slide under both low and high power. Draw, label, and describe your findings. Describe how it appears differently from the healthy lung slide.

TM _____

Slide name _____

Description _____

_____

_____

_____

_____

4. Identify the following structures on the trachea slide under both low and high power. Draw, label, and describe your findings in the spaces provided.
   - Ciliated pseudostratified columnar epithelium
   - Goblet cell
   - Hyaline cartilage

TM _____

Slide name _____

Description _____

_____

_____

_____

_____

TM _____

Slide name _____

Description _____

_____

_____

_____

_____

Activity Questions

1. What is the difference between a terminal bronchiole and a respiratory bronchiole?

_____

_____

_____

2. What do goblet cells secrete? How does the secretion work together with the cilia to protect the lungs?

_____

_____

_____

_____

3. Critical Thinking: Name the type of epithelium that composes the alveoli. Based on the function of the lungs, why does that type of tissue make sense?

_____

_____

_____

4. **Critical Thinking:** A common theme throughout the text is that structure equals function. Compare the structure of the normal lung with that of the carcinogenic lung. How do you think that the function of the lung is changed because of the structural change?

_____

_____

_____

_____

Activity 21-4

Body Mapping: Respiratory System

This activity is similar to other body mapping assignments that you have done in the past. However, you will be starting from scratch for this mapping assignment and will use your body map for several more activities this semester.

Activity Instructions

Work with another member of the class on this activity. Use Figures 13-4, 13-5, 13-6, and 13-7 in the textbook to help you with your drawings.

1. Cut two large pieces of butcher paper as long as each of you are tall. Have one person lie down on one piece of paper. This person must lie supine, legs slightly apart, head facing to the right.

2. The other person, using a black marker, must trace the outline of the person lying down with the head turned to the side, including the nose. The head and neck represent a midsagittal plane and the body drawing represents a frontal plane.

3. Now switch places so that you will have two body maps.

4. Roll up one body map to be used in Activity 23-3.

5. Follow the instructions for steps 6 through 20 to create your respiratory system body map. Use a pencil to start with; when you are satisfied with your drawing, use the color markers as indicated in the instructions. As you create your body map, use Table 21.4 to keep track of the color and number assigned to each structure.

Table 21.4 Respiratory System Body Map

Name of Structure	Corresponding Color	Corresponding Number on Body Map
Diaphragm		
Epiglottis		
Hard palate		
Inferior nasal concha		
Larynx		
Left lung		
Lobar bronchi		
Mainstem bronchi		
Middle nasal concha		
Nasopharynx		
Oropharynx		
Palatine tonsil		
Pharyngeal tonsil		
Right lung		
Soft palate		
Superior nasal concha		
Thyroid cartilage		
Trachea		

The structures in steps 6 through 11 are drawn in a midsagittal plane.

6. Draw a thick, curved line separating the nasal cavity from the oral cavity to represent the **soft** and **hard palates.**

7. Draw the **superior, middle,** and **inferior nasal conchae** in the nasal cavity.

8. Draw a tube extending from the nasal cavity inferiorly to slightly above the level of the chin. Label the three regions of this tube (**nasopharynx, oropharynx,** and **laryngopharynx**).

9. Draw collections of dots to represent the **pharyngeal tonsil** and **palatine tonsil.**

10. Draw a slender tube (the esophagus) that extends inferiorly from the laryngopharynx.

11. Draw a second tube (about 2 in long) descending from the laryngopharynx, anterior to the esophagus. This tube represents the **larynx**. Label the **thyroid cartilage** on the larynx.

12. Draw a flap that extends superiorly from the larynx toward the palatine tonsil. This flap represents the **epiglottis.**

The rest of the structures are drawn in a frontal plane.

13. Draw a tube about 4 in. long extending inferiorly from the larynx. This is the **trachea.**

14. Draw in a muscular flap (or dome) between the thoracic and abdominal cavities; this is the **diaphragm.**

15. Draw two tubes branching left and right from the end of the trachea. These are the **mainstem (primary) bronchi.**

16. Draw the **right** and **left lungs**, including the horizontal fissure on the right lung. Be sure to have the lungs extend down to the diaphragm.

17. Draw the **lobar bronchi** extending to each lobe of the lung. Be sure to draw three lobar bronchi on the right lung and two on the left lung.

18. Trace over the structures above, using different color markers (any color except for **blue** and **purple**). Write the color code in the table above.

19. Trace over the surface of the lung with a **blue** marker.

20. Leave a space and draw a corresponding tracing of the lung with a **purple** marker.

21. Quiz your lab partner to identify the organs and structures that you just drew, using your answer key to make sure that the answers are correct.

Activity Questions

1. Which layer of the lung's serous membrane does the blue line represent?

_____

2. Which layer of the lung's serous membrane does the purple line represent?

_____

3. What is the space between the membranes called and what is found in that space?

_____

Post-Lab Assessment

1. List the conducting zone structures in the order in which air passes through them.

_____

_____

_____

2. List the respiratory zone structures in the order in which air passes through them.

_____

_____

_____

3. Name the C-shaped rings of connective tissue strengthening the trachea. Describe how the components of the connective tissue contribute to the structure of the trachea.

_____

_____

_____

4. Describe the locations of the serous membranes that surround the lungs. Describe the function of the serous membranes.

_____

_____

_____

5. **Critical Thinking:** Jade went to the physician complaining of congestion and watery eyes. The physician tapped under Jade's eyes and on her forehead and pinched the bridge of her nose. What was the physician assessing?

_____

_____

_____

Respiratory System Physiology

Textbook Correlation: Chapter 13—The Respiratory System

Details

Activities	Activity Objectives	Required Materials	Estimated Time
22-1: Pleural Fluid Function	Demonstrate and explain the function of pleural fluid	● Four glass slides ● One squirt bottle filled with water	10 min
22-2: Pulmonary Ventilation	Demonstrate and explain the pressure/volume relationship that occurs during pulmonary ventilation; relate the pressure/volume changes to inspiration and expiration	● Functional lung model	15 min
22-3: Sheep or Pig Pluck Dissection	Identify the parts of a sheep/pig pluck; observe inflation and deflation of the lungs; determine why lungs float when placed in water	● Sheep or pig pluck ● Dissecting tray ● Gloves ● Scalpel ● Measuring tape ● Beaker	25 min

Details (Continued)

Activities	Activity Objectives	Required Materials	Estimated Time
22-4: Spirometry—Measuring Lung Volumes and Capacities	Demonstrate your ability to use a spirometer and interpret the data collected; determine respiratory volumes and capacities; apply the data obtained from the spirometer to determine additional lung volumes	<ul><li>Spirometer</li><li>Mouthpiece</li><li>Bleach container</li></ul>	40 min

Overview

You have most likely seen an elderly individual who is wheelchair-bound and connected to an oxygen tank. Perhaps you've wondered why the person needs a tank of oxygen when oxygen is abundant in the environment. In most cases, the answer is that the person's pulmonary ventilation is insufficient because of lung damage from exposure to harmful irritants, years of smoking, or infection. In the last lab, you learned that gas exchange occurs in the alveoli, which you saw represented on a model and under the microscope. In patients with chronic obstructive pulmonary disease (COPD), the alveolar or bronchial structure has changed, which makes it harder to bring in sufficient amounts of oxygen and to expel enough carbon dioxide. COPD and some other respiratory diseases can be diagnosed by a procedure called *spirometry*, which measures various lung volumes and capacities. Today's lab activities focus on the mechanism of pulmonary ventilation and measuring lung volumes and capacities in healthy individuals.

Need to Know

- **Pleural membranes:** serous membranes that enclose the lungs
  - **Parietal pleura:** the most superficial membrane that lines the rib cage and the superior portion of the diaphragm
  - **Visceral pleura:** deep membrane that directly covers the surface of the lungs
  - **Pleural cavity:** fluid-filled space between the two pleural membranes; the fluid anchors the pleurae together

- **Boyle's law:**
  - Explains the relationship between pressure and volume
  - For a given number of gas (or liquid) molecules:
    - As the container volume increases, the pressure decreases.
    - As the container volume decreases, the gas pressure increases.
  - Think about squeezing a tube of toothpaste from the bottom. Decreasing the tube volume increases pressure, forcing toothpaste out of the tube.

- **Pulmonary ventilation:** the mechanical process of moving air in and out of the lungs
  - **Inspiration:**
    - The **volume** of the lungs increases owing to the action of the:
      - **Diaphragm:** a dome-shaped muscle that flattens and moves inferiorly
      - **External intercostals:** muscles that expand the rib cage laterally and the sternum anteriorly
    - The **pressure** of the thoracic cavity decreases below atmospheric pressure
      - Air enters the lungs until the intrapulmonary pressure equals atmospheric pressure
  - **Expiration:**
    - The **volume** of the lungs decreases because of the recoil of the inspiratory muscles and lung tissue
    - The **pressure** of the lungs increases above atmospheric pressure
      - Air exits the lungs until the intrapulmonary pressure equals the atmospheric pressure
      - **Forced** expiration requires muscle action from the abdominals and internal intercostals to decrease lung volume to a greater extent

- **Volumes** and **Capacities:**
  - **Tidal volume (TV):** the amount of air that moves in and out of the lungs (both conduction and respiratory zones) with each breath (approximately 500 mL)
  - **Minute ventilation:** the amount of air that moves in and out of the lungs in one minute
    - Respirations per minute × tidal volume
    - Does not take into account the **anatomical dead space**
      - Trapped air in the conducting zone (approximately 30% of tidal volume)—location of no gas exchange
  - **Alveolar ventilation rate (AVR):** much more effective respiration value than minute value
    - AVR = [tidal volume – dead space (tidal volume × 0.3)] × respiration rate
  - **Expiratory reserve volume (ERV):** the amount of air that can be forcibly expelled after a normal expiration
  - **Vital capacity (VC):** the total amount of exchangeable air
    - Vital capacity = tidal volume + inspiratory reserve volume + expiratory reserve volume
  - **Inspiratory reserve volume (IRV):** amount of additional air that can be inhaled after a normal tidal volume respiration
    - Calculated by the following formula:

$$\text{IRV} = \text{Average VC} - (\text{average TV} + \text{average ERV})$$

Pre-Lab Activity

Students should complete this activity before completing the lab activities that follow.

1. Label the parietal pleura, the visceral pleura, and the intrapleural cavity on the diagram below.

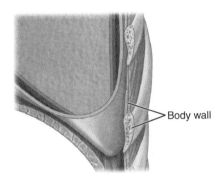

Body wall

2. Label the following terms on the figure below:
   - Expiratory reserve volume
   - Inspiratory reserve volume
   - Tidal volume
   - Vital capacity

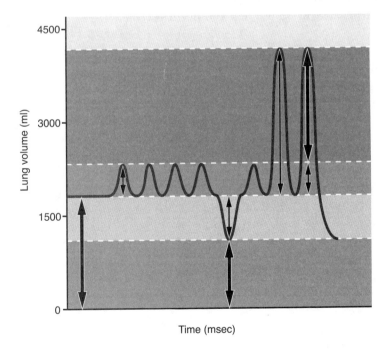

Pleural Fluid Function

This activity uses two glass slides to represent the two layers of the pleurae and water to represent the pleural fluid.

Activity Instructions and Questions

1. Obtain two glass slides and place them on top of one another. Try to pull the two slides apart. Does it require much strength to do this?

_____

_____

2. Get a squirt bottle filled with water. Separate the two slides used above and put a few drops of water on one of them. Place the second slide on top of the first slide. Try to pull the two slides apart. Can you do it? Is it easy? Now slide the two surfaces across one another. Describe what happens.

_____

_____

_____

3. Get two new glass slides. Pour many drops of water on one slide and place the second slide on top of the first. Try to pull the slides apart. Can you do it? Does it require much strength to pull them apart?

_____

_____

_____

4. Which of the above scenarios do you think most accurately represents the amount of pleural fluid in the pleural space in a healthy individual? Explain why your answer is correct and why the other possibilities are incorrect.

_____

_____

_____

_____

_____

Activity 22-2

Pulmonary Ventilation

This activity uses a lung model to investigate the pressure/volume differences that occur during pulmonary ventilation. In this model, the balloons represent the lungs and the rubber diaphragm represents the muscular diaphragm.

Activity Instructions and Questions

1. Work in groups of two; one person should follow the instructions while the other writes down observations.

2. Pull the rubber diaphragm located on the bell jar. Fill in the first row of Table 22.1. (Use the Need to Know section as well.)

3. Push the rubber diaphragm in and record your observations in the second row of the table.

Table 22.1 Lung Model Data

	Size (Volume) of Balloon (↑ or ↓)	Volume in "Cavity" (↑ or ↓)	Pressure in "Cavity" (↑ or ↓)	Similar to Expiration or Inspiration?
Pull rubber diaphragm				
Push rubber diaphragm				

4. Based on your observations above, what is the relationship between volume and pressure in the thoracic cavity during pulmonary ventilation? Cite an example from the activity observations.

_____

_____

_____

_____

_____

5. Does the volume of the balloon increase or decrease during expiration? Explain your answer.

_____

_____

_____

_____

Sheep or Pig Pluck Dissection

In this activity, you will explore respiratory system anatomy using a sheep or pig pluck, which is a collection of organs. The plucks used today will contain respiratory system organs. (To see additional dissection images, visit the text's online site and view the Dissection Atlas.)

Activity Instructions

1. Put on gloves. Obtain a dissecting tray, scalpel, and measuring tape.

2. Obtain a sheep or pig pluck and place it on the dissecting tray.

3. Touch the lungs, making note of the texture. Use the measuring tape to measure the width and length of the lungs. Answer Activity Questions 1 through 3.

4. Identify the following structures on the sheep pluck:
   - Larynx (if visible)
   - Trachea with cartilage rings
   - Bronchi (right and left)
   - Right and left lobar bronchi
   - Pulmonary arteries and veins (if visible)
   - Diaphragm (if attached)

5. Inflate the sheep lungs by placing a piece of tubing down the trachea and connecting the other end to a gas outlet or foot air pump. Turn on the gas or pump the foot pump to inflate the lungs. Observe the lungs deflate. (**Safety Note:** Do NOT inflate the tube with your mouth!)

6. Cut a small section of the lung and place it in a beaker filled two thirds full of water. Answer the rest of the Activity Questions.

Activity Questions

1. Describe how the lungs feel in your hands.

_____

_____

_____

2. Record the length and width of the lungs. How do you think the lungs compare in size with those of adult human lungs?

_____

_____

3. Name the membrane that directly touches the surface of the lung.

_____

4. Did the lungs float or sink when you placed them in the water?

_____

5. Air weighs less than water. Based on this statement, explain your observation from question 4.

_____

_____

_____

_____

6. **Critical Thinking:** How do you think the results in question 4 would be different if the lungs had never been inflated? Explain your answer.

_____

_____

_____

_____

Spirometry—Measuring Lung Volumes and Capacities

This activity will enable you to measure your own (or your partner's) lung function using a **spirometer**—a piece of equipment that contains a barrel of water and a mouthpiece. As the subject blows into the mouthpiece, the exhaled air displaces the water in the barrel, and the amount of water displaced represents the amount of exhaled air.

Activity Instructions

Work in groups of two. Keep in mind that this piece of equipment ONLY measures the amount of exhaled air (not inhaled air). When prompted, record the readings in Table 22.2.

1. Check the machine to determine the units that the machine measures (liters [L] or milliliters [mL]).

2. Choose one person to be the subject. Instruct the subject to sit still and breathe normally. The test administrator should read all of the instructions prior to collecting the data.

3. Instruct the subject to close his or her eyes and to breathe normally while holding the mouthpiece. On the fifth inhale, instruct the subject to bring the mouthpiece to the mouth and exhale normally into the mouthpiece. The subject should not force air out during the exhale. Record the value, which is the **tidal volume (TV),** in the table below. Tell the subject to repeat this two more times, record the values, and calculate the average of the tidal volume values.

4. Tell the subject to breathe normally and then insert the mouthpiece after a normal exhale. Instruct the subject to empty his or her lungs as much as possible and record the value. This is the **expiratory reserve volume (ERV).** The subject should repeat this two times and the average should be recorded.

5. Instruct the subject to inhale as deeply as possible, insert the mouthpiece, and exhale as much as possible. Coach the subject to inhale and exhale very deeply—a valid reading for this activity requires significant effort! Record this value as the **vital capacity (VC).** Repeat two more times and calculate the average VC value.

6. The **inspiratory reserve volume (IRV)** cannot be determined by the spirometer, but it can be mathematically calculated using this formula:

$$IRV = \text{average VC} - (\text{average TV} + \text{average ERV})$$

7. Place the mouthpiece in the bleach container.

Table 22.2 Spirometry Data				
	Tidal Volume	Expiratory Reserve Volume	Vital Capacity	Inspiratory Reserve Volume
Trial 1				
Trial 2				
Trial 3				
Average				

Activity Questions

Record all values in correct units.

1. Ask your instructor for a copy of a nomogram chart to determine if your vital capacity is within the normal range. Find your age and height on the chart (round off if necessary) and follow your age down and your height across; your normal vital capacity is where your age and height intersect. Is your vital capacity within the normal range for your height and weight? If not, describe some factors that could result in a smaller or larger vital capacity.

   _____

   _____

   _____

2. Determine the **minute ventilation** of the subject. Count the subject's number of respirations per minute. Record the number of respirations in 1 minute:

   _____

   Multiply the number of respirations by tidal volume to calculate the minute ventilation.

   _____

3. Determine the value of the subject's **anatomical dead space,** which is approximately 30% of the tidal volume (tidal volume $\times$ 0.3).

   _____

4. The **alveolar ventilation rate (AVR)** is a more accurate measurement of the effectiveness of respiration. Use this formula to calculate the AVR:

   $$AVR = (\text{tidal volume} - \text{dead space}) \times \text{respiratory rate}$$

   _____

5. Which muscles were recruited (used) when the ERV was measured but did not participate in the determination of the tidal volume?

_____

6. Is the subject a smoker?

_____

7. If the subject is a smoker, compare the results of spirometry with those of a nonsmoker. If the subject is a nonsmoker, compare the results with those of a smoker. Describe the differences in spirometry results between a smoker and a nonsmoker. If possible, compare results between subjects of similar age and height.

_____

_____

_____

_____

_____

_____

8. What are some other factors (besides smoking) that can alter tidal volume and AVR?

_____

_____

_____

_____

_____

_____

Post-Lab Assessment

1. Describe the importance of pleural fluid.

_____

_____

_____

_____

_____

2. Describe the changes in pressure and volume in the lungs at the beginning of inspiration. Does air enter the lungs or leave the lungs during inspiration? Why? When does inspiration stop?

_____

_____

_____

_____

_____

_____

Match the following terms with the correct definition. Not all terms will be used.

A. Alveolar ventilation rate
B. Anatomical dead space
C. Boyle's law
D. Expiration
E. Expiratory reserve volume
F. Inspiration
G. Inspiratory reserve volume
H. Minute ventilation
I. Tidal volume
J. Vital capacity

3. Amount of air that moves in and out of the conduction and respiratory zones during one breath: _____

4. Law that states that the pressure of a gas is inversely related to volume of the container that contains the gas: _____

5. Location in which air is trapped and no gas exchange takes place: _____

6. The amount of air that enters and exits the lungs in 1 minute: _____

7. The amount of air that is forcibly exhaled after a normal exhalation: _____

8. The phase of ventilation during which lung volume decreases: _____

9. The total amount of air exchanged in a normal respiration plus the amount that can be forcibly inhaled and exhaled: _____

10. A more accurate indication of pulmonary effectiveness than minute volume because it takes fresh air intake into account: _____

23

Digestive System Anatomy

Textbook Correlation: Chapter 14—The Digestive System

Details

Activities	Activity Objectives	Required Materials	Estimated Time
23-1: Gastrointestinal Tract Anatomy	Identify the organs of the GI tract; identify the structures found in each organ	• Midsagittal head model • Frontal head model • Stomach model • Small intestine model • Large intestine model	30 min
23-2: Accessory Organs	Identify the accessory organs of the digestive system; identify the structures found in the accessory organs	• Midsagittal head model • Teeth model(s) • Liver model • Gallbladder model • Pancreas model	25 min
23-3: Body Mapping— Digestive System	Draw and identify the organs of the digestive system	• Body map from Exercise 21-4 • Markers (20 + colors)	45 min
23-4: Digestive System Histology	Identify the organs microscopically; identify the layers of the organ walls microscopically	• Histology wall models • Microscope Slides: esophagus– stomach junction, small intestine, large intestine, rectoanal junction, pancreas, liver	50 min
23-5: Digestive System Dissection (Optional)	Identify the organs of the digestive system in a specimen	• Digestive tract from cow or pig • Dissection tray • Gloves • Measuring tape	30 min

Overview

The last time that you went to an amusement park, did you go on a "rushing rapids" ride? Imagine this scenario: You first travel down a narrow canal in anticipation of the ride ahead. Next, you hit a large patch of very rough water that really rocks the inner tube (and its contents!). Then the river slows down a bit and bystanders can pay some money to shoot water guns at you. Twists and turns ensue as you follow a tortuous route down the river. Finally, the river widens as your inner tube travels up an incline and across a platform, where you unload and exit the ride.

That ride is similar to what occurs in the digestive system. Loading onto the ride from the dock is similar to putting food in your mouth. The narrow canal is similar to food traveling down the esophagus. The stomach, with its muscular layers, pummels food just as you were pummeled by the rough waters. Getting water squirted at you is similar to events that occur in the duodenum (proximal segment of the small intestine): the "bystanders" in the digestive system are the pancreas, liver, and gallbladder, which "shoot" their secretions through ducts into the duodenum. The twist and turns are analogous to the coils of the rest of the small intestine. Traveling up and across is similar to the movement in the large intestine (except that the feces will also travel down), and exiting the ride is similar to the feces leaving the anus (defacation).

Need to Know

Gastrointestinal Tract

- **Oral cavity:** opening through which food is ingested
  - **Lips:** help to keep food in the oral cavity
  - **Palate:** soft and hard palates separate the oral cavity from the nasal cavity

- **Pharynx:** a muscular tube that extends from the nasal cavity down the throat

- **Esophagus:** a long muscular tube inferior to the laryngopharynx
  - Propels the bolus (food) inferiorly through the thoracic cavity and the diaphragm

- **Stomach:** a large muscular organ that holds food and breaks it down mechanically
  - Composed of these regions:
    - **Cardia:** where the esophagus connects to the stomach; a slender ring
    - **Fundus:** large "bump" located laterally and superiorly to the cardia
    - **Body:** largest, broadest region of the stomach
    - **Pylorus:** inferior to the body; a slender portion that connects to the small intestine
      - Regulates the amount of food that can enter the small intestine

- **Small intestine:** long, winding tube located in the inferior portion of the abdominal cavity
  - Regions from proximal to distal:
    - **Duodenum:** receives food from the pyloric region of the stomach; most digestion occurs here
    - **Jejunum**
    - **Ileum:** delivers food to the large intestine

- **Large intestine:** larger-diameter tube connecting the small intestine to the anus
  - Regions:
    - **Cecum:** receives undigested material from the ileum
      - **Ileocecal valve:** regulates the amount of material that enters the cecum

○ **Ascending colon** on the right side, which extends vertically from the cecum
   ■ **Hepatic flexure:** curved, most superior portion of the ascending colon
○ **Transverse colon:** horizontal portion of the large intestine, which connects the ascending and descending segments
   ■ **Splenic flexure:** curve on the left side of the colon
○ **Descending colon:** vertical region located on the left side of the organ
○ **Sigmoid colon:** S-shaped tube that extends from the descending colon
● **Rectum:** straight, vertical, short tube
● **Anal canal:** last and shortest part of the large intestine
   ○ **Anus:** opening to the external environment
      ■ **Internal anal sphincter:** involuntary smooth muscle
      ■ **External anal sphincter:** voluntary skeletal muscle

Histology of the Gastrointestinal Organ Wall

● **Mucosa:** surrounds the lumen (space) of the organ
   ● Composed of:
      ○ Epithelial tissue (surrounding the lumen)
         ■ Nonkeratinized stratified squamous epithelium in the oropharynx, laryngopharynx, esophagus, and anus
         ■ Simple columnar epithelium in the stomach and intestines
         ■ Embedded with mucus-producing **goblet cells**
      ○ Lamina propria (areolar connective tissue)

● **Submucosa:** external to the mucosa
   ● Composed of dense connective tissue

● **Muscularis externa:** surrounds the submucosa
   ● Composed of smooth muscle arranged in layers
      ○ **Circular** smooth muscle layer (inner layer)
      ○ **Longitudinal** smooth muscle layer (outer layer)

● **Serosa: Peritoneal** membrane that surrounds the organs

● Unique modifications:
   ● **Stomach:** modifications enhance digestion
      ○ Extra **oblique** smooth muscle layer
      ○ **Gastric glands** secrete hydrogen ions, pepsinogen, intrinsic factor, and hormones
   ● **Small intestine:** modifications increase surface area for absorption
      ○ **Circular folds:** large folds in the mucosa and submucosa of the organ wall
      ○ **Villi:** folds in the epithelium
      ○ **Microvilli:** tiny hairlike folds in the cell membrane of the epithelial cells
   ● **Large intestine:**
      ○ **Teniae coli:** longitudinal muscle layer
      ○ **Haustra:** bulges that result from the contraction of the teniae coli

Accessory Organs

- **Tongue:** large skeletal muscle located in the oral cavity

- **Teeth:**
  - Types:
    - ○ **Incisors:** two front teeth
    - ○ **Cuspids (canines):** lateral to incisors; "vampire" teeth
    - ○ **Bicuspids (premolars):** two points per tooth
    - ○ **Molars:** four to five points per tooth
  - Parts of a tooth:
    - ○ Entire tooth can be divided into two parts
      - ■ **Crown:** visible portion of the tooth
      - ■ **Root:** embeds the tooth into the bone
    - ○ **Dentin** (hard connective tissue) makes up most of the structure of the tooth
      - ■ Dentin in the crown is covered with a hard white surface called **enamel**
      - ■ Dentin in the root is surrounded by **cementum** and connected to the bone by **periodontal ligaments**
    - ○ **Pulp cavity:** space in the center of the tooth that contains the **pulp**
      - ■ Rich with blood vessels, nerves, and lymphatics
      - ■ Extends down the tooth root as a **root canal**

- **Salivary glands:**
  - **Parotid glands, submandibular glands,** and **sublingual glands**

- **Liver:** located in the upper right quadrant
  - Produces bile, detoxifies blood, produces blood proteins, and performs important metabolic roles
  - Contains right, left, quadrate, and caudate lobes
  - **Lobules:** hexagonal structural and functional units of the liver
    - ○ Contain numerous **hepatocytes,** or liver cells
    - ○ **Central vein:** located in the center of a lobule
  - **Portal triads:** located at the corners of lobules
    - ○ **Hepatic artery branch:** supplies the **hepatocytes** (liver cells) with oxygen
    - ○ **Hepatic portal vein:** delivers newly obtained nutrient-rich blood to the liver from the digestive system organs
    - ○ **Bile duct:** drains freshly made bile from the hepatocytes toward the right and left hepatic ducts

- **Gallbladder:** small green tear-shaped storage organ for bile
  - Located on the inferior surface of the liver

- **Pancreas:** exocrine (digestive enzymes) and endocrine gland (insulin, glucagon)
  - Located inferiorly and posteriorly to the stomach and to the left of the duodenum

- **Duct system:** series of ducts that deliver bile from the liver and gallbladder and digestive enzymes from the pancreas to the duodenum
  - **Right** and **left hepatic ducts:** receive bile from the bile ducts of the portal triad
  - **Common hepatic duct** created by the merger of the right and left hepatic ducts
  - **Cystic duct:** supplies and drains bile from the gallbladder
  - **Common bile duct** created by the merger of the common hepatic duct and cystic duct
    - ○ Brings bile toward the duodenum
  - **Pancreatic duct:** large duct that extends horizontally across the pancreas
    - ○ Brings pancreatic enzymes toward the duodenum
  - **Hepatopancreatic ampulla** created by the merger of the pancreatic duct and the common bile duct; deposits bile and pancreatic enzymes into the duodenum
    - ○ **Hepatopancreatic sphincter:** muscle that regulates the amount of fluid that can enter the duodenum from the hepatopancreatic ampulla

Pre-Lab Activity

Students should complete this activity before completing the lab activities that follow.

Use the terms in the Need to Know section to complete this assignment.

1. Fill in the labels on the illustration below.

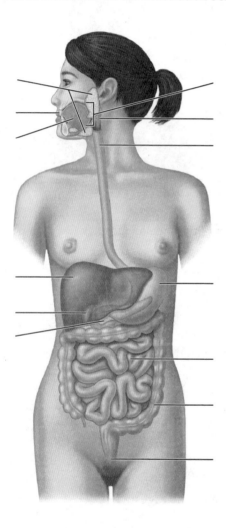

2. Color the layers of the organ wall according to the color scheme below:
   - Mucosa: red
   - Submucosa: green
   - Circular smooth muscle layer: purple
   - Longitudinal smooth muscle layer: orange
   - Serosa: blue

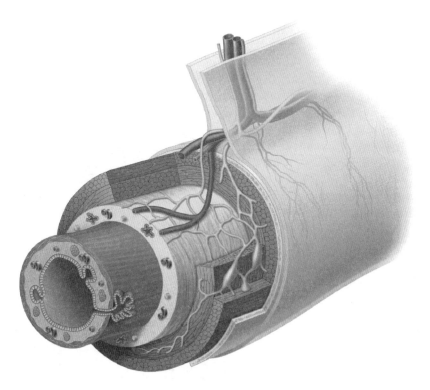

3. Color the accessory organs according to the color scheme listed below:
   - Liver: brown
   - Gallbladder: green
   - Pancreas: red
   - Duodenum: purple

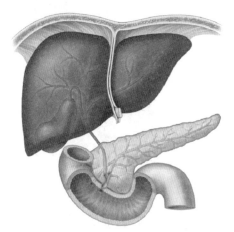

4. The digestive system contains many glands. Think back to when you studied tissue. What general type of tissue makes up all glands?

_____

Gastrointestinal Tract Anatomy

Activity Instructions

On the midsagittal head and torso models, identify the organs and structures listed in the left-hand column of Table 23.1. As you identify each structure, write down the corresponding number in the right-hand column. Name the model that you used to identify each organ or structure in the middle column. Refer to Figures 14-4, 14-9, 14-13, 14-16, and 14-23 in the textbook.

Table 23.1 Gastrointestinal Tract Anatomy		
Organ or Structure	**Model**	**Corresponding Number on the Model**
Oral cavity		
Lips		
Hard palate		
Soft palate		
Pharynx		
Oropharynx		
Laryngopharynx		
Esophagus		
Stomach		
Cardia		

Table 23.1 Gastrointestinal Tract Anatomy (continued)

Organ or Structure	Model	Corresponding Number on the Model
Fundus		
Body		
Pylorus		
Pyloric sphincter		
Greater curvature		
Lesser curvature		
Rugae		
Oblique smooth muscle layer		
Circular smooth muscle layer		
Longitudinal smooth muscle layer		
Small intestine		
Duodenum		
Jejunum		
Ileum		
Circular folds		
Greater omentum (part of the peritoneum)		

(continued)

Table 23.1	Gastrointestinal Tract Anatomy (continued)	
Organ or Structure	**Model**	**Corresponding Number on the Model**
Large intestine		
Cecum		
Ileocecal valve		
Ascending (right) colon		
Hepatic flexure		
Transverse colon		
Splenic flexure		
Descending (left) colon		
Sigmoid colon		
Rectum		
Anal canal		
Anus		
Teniae coli		
Haustra		
Internal anal sphincter		
External anal sphincter		

Activity Questions

1. Once the food (bolus) enters the laryngopharynx, where does it go? What structure prevents it from entering the larynx?

_____

_____

2. Name the unique muscle layer found in the stomach. Based on the function of the stomach, why do you think that an additional muscle layer is found in the wall of the stomach?

_____

_____

_____

3. The wall of the small intestine is modified for one of its major functions: absorption. What modification of the intestinal wall is visible to the naked eye that increases the surface area for absorption of nutrients?

_____

_____

4. The large intestine has long, longitudinal, parallel strips of muscle that contract to form bulges in the organ wall. Name the muscle and the resulting bulges.

_____

_____

5. Name the most superficial muscle surrounding the anus.

_____

_____

Accessory Organs

Activity Instructions

On the midsagittal head, teeth, and torso models, identify the organs and structures listed in the left-hand column of Table 23.2. As you identify each structure, write down the corresponding number in the right-hand column. Name the model that you used to identify each organ or structure in the middle column. Refer to Figures 14-9, 14-10, 14-11, 14-18, and 14-19 in the textbook.

Table 23.2 Accessory Organs		
Organ or Structure	**Model**	**Corresponding Number on the Model**
Tongue		
Teeth		
Incisors		
Cuspids (canines)		
Premolars (bicuspids)		
Molars		
Crown		
Root		
Pulp cavity		

Table 23.2 Accessory Organs (continued)

Organ or Structure	Model	Corresponding Number on the Model
Root canal		
Dentin		
Enamel		
Cementum		
Salivary glands		
Parotid glands		
Sublingual gland		
Submandibular glands		
Pancreas		
Pancreatic duct		
Liver		
Right lobe		
Left lobe		
Caudate lobe		
Quadrate lobe		
Falciform ligament		
Hepatic artery		

(continued)

Table 23.2	Accessory Organs (continued)	
Organ or Structure	**Model**	**Corresponding Number on the Model**
Hepatic portal vein		
Hepatic vein		
Inferior vena cava		
Gallbladder		
Bile ducts		
Hepatic ducts (right and left)		
Common hepatic duct		
Cystic duct		
Common bile duct		
Hepatopancreatic ampulla		

Activity Questions

1. Name the hard, white part of a tooth that contains calcium.

_____

2. Name the part of the tooth that is embedded in the alveoli (spaces) of the mandible and maxillae.

_____

3. Describe the flow of blood through the hepatic portal system.

_____

_____

_____

4. Name the gland located below the tongue.

_____

5. Name the duct that directly drains the gallbladder.

_____

Activity 23-3

Body Mapping: Digestive System

Activity Instructions

Use your unmarked body map (frontal view, with the head turned to the side) from Activity 21-4 to make a body map of the digestive system. Work in groups of two.

Draw the following structures in pencil until you are satisfied with your drawings.

1. Draw a thick, curved line separating the nasal cavity from the oral cavity to represent the **soft** and **hard palates.**

2. Draw the **tongue, lips,** and two **teeth** in the **oral cavity.**

3. Draw a tube extending from the oral cavity inferiorly to slightly above the level of the chin. This tube represents the **oropharynx** and **laryngopharynx.**

4. Draw a slender tube extending inferiorly from the laryngopharynx. This tube represents the **esophagus.** Stop about halfway in the thoracic cavity.

5. Draw in a muscular flap between the thoracic and abdominal cavities; this is the **diaphragm.** (Although not a digestive system organ, it makes an excellent reference point for digestive system organs.)

6. Return to the esophagus in the thoracic cavity. Continue drawing it in a frontal plane inferiorly. Use a **dotted line** to represent the esophagus once you enter the abdominal cavity. The dotted line represents the fact that it is located posterior to the liver.

7. Draw the **liver** in the upper right quadrant. Be sure that the liver extends over the esophagus.

8. Draw the **gallbladder** on the liver using **dotted lines.** This represents the location of the gallbladder.

9. Draw the **stomach** in the upper left quadrant, using **dotted lines** to represent the portion that is deep to the liver.

10. Draw the **pancreas** in with **dotted lines** to represent that is located posterior to the stomach.

11. Draw the **duodenum** extending slightly laterally and inferiorly from the stomach.

12. Draw the **large intestine,** including the flexures (hepatic and splenic) and sigmoid colon.

13. Add the **rectum** and **anus** to your drawing.

14. Draw the coils of the **small intestine** between the right and left segments of the large intestine.

15. Once you are satisfied with your drawings, draw over the organs with markers. Use the key in the table below to determine the correct color for each organ.

16. Give each organ or region by giving each a number on the body map and write the corresponding number in Table 23.3. Use the body map and table to quiz one another.

Table 23.3   Body Map Key

Organ	Corresponding Color	Corresponding Number on Body Map
Anus	Purple	
Ascending colon	Black	
Descending colon	Peach	
Duodenum	Gray	
Esophagus	Teal	
Gallbladder	Green	
Hard palate	Dark green	
Ileum	Light blue	
Jejunum	Magenta	
Lips	Red	
Liver	Brown	
Nasopharynx	Light pink	

Table 23.3   Body Map Key (continued)

Organ	Corresponding Color	Corresponding Number on Body Map
Oral cavity	(no color)	
Oropharynx	Light gray	
Pancreas	Yellow	
Rectum	Light brown	
Sigmoid colon	Orange	
Soft palate	Light green	
Stomach	Pink	
Teeth	(no color)	
Tongue	Navy (dark) blue	
Transverse colon	Blue	

Activity 23-4

Digestive System Histology

Studying the histology of the digestive organs will help you understand the complex functions of this system.

Activity Instructions

Identify the following microscopic structures of the digestive system. Draw and label your findings. Note: It is best to look at the model(s) of the GI tract wall if available. Refer to Figures 14-14, 14-17, 14-18 and 14-20 in the textbook.

1. Identify the following structures on the esophagus slide under low power. Draw, label, and describe your findings.
   - Nonkeratinized stratified squamous epithelium
   - Smooth muscle

TM _____

Slide name _____

Description _____

_____

_____

_____

_____

2. Identify the following structures on the stomach slide using both low and high power. Draw, label, and describe your findings.
   - Mucosa
     - Epithelium
     - Lamina propria
     - Gastric pits
   - Submucosa
     - Submucosal glands
   - Muscularis externa

TM _____

Slide name _____

Description _____

_____

_____

_____

_____

TM _____

Slide name _____

Description _____

_____

_____

_____

3. Identify the following structures on the small intestine slide using both low and high power. Draw, label, and describe your findings.

- Mucosa
  - Villi
  - Epithelium
    - ○ Microvilli
  - Goblet cells
  - Lamina propria
    - ○ Peyer's patches (may be seen extending into the submucosa)
- Submucosa
  - Submucosal glands
- Muscularis externa

TM _____

Slide name _____

Description _____

_____

_____

_____

TM _____

Slide name _____

Description _____

_____

_____

_____

4. Identify the following structures on the large intestine slide under both low and high power. Draw, label, and describe your findings.

- Mucosa
  - Intestinal crypts
  - Epithelium
  - Goblet cells
  - Lamina propria
- Submucosa
- Muscularis externa

TM _____

Slide name _____

Description _____

_____

_____

_____

_____

TM _____

Slide name _____

Description _____

_____

_____

_____

_____

5. Identify the following structures on the rectoanal junction slide using low power. Draw, label, and describe your findings.
   ● Mucosa
     ● Epithelium
     ● Lamina propria

TM _____

Slide name _____

Description _____

_____

_____

_____

_____

6. Identify the following structures on the pancreas slide, using low power. Draw, label, and describe your findings.
   ● Acini
   ● Pancreatic islets

TM _____

Slide name _____

Description _____

_____

_____

_____

_____

7. Identify the following structures on the liver slide using both low and high power. Draw, label, and describe your findings.
- Lobule
- Central vein
- Portal triad
  - Hepatic artery branch
  - Hepatic portal vein
  - Bile duct

TM _____

Slide name _____

Description _____

_____

_____

_____

_____

TM _____

Slide name _____

Description _____

_____

_____

_____

_____

Activity Questions

1. How does the epithelium change at the esophagus–stomach junction? Why do you think that the type of epithelium changes (based on the function of each organ)?

_____

_____

_____

_____

2. Name the type of epithelial tissue that lines most of the GI tract (stomach to rectum).

_____

3. How does the epithelium change at the rectoanal junction? Why do you think that the type of epithelium changes?

_____

_____

_____

4. Which secretory portion of the pancreas is considered exocrine?

_____

5. How does the epithelium differ between the hepatic artery branch and the bile duct?

_____

_____

6. The liver and pancreas are both glands. Name the general type of tissue that makes up both organs.

_____

7. **Critical Thinking:** The lamina propria is composed of areolar connective tissue. Why does it make sense that this is part of the mucosal layer, supporting epithelial tissue? Hint: Think back to epithelial tissue characteristics and areolar connective tissue.

_____

_____

_____

8. **Critical Thinking:** Goblet cells secrete mucus. Why does it make sense that the distal portion of the small intestine and the large intestine contain lots of these cells?

_____

_____

_____

_____

Activity 23-5

Digestive System Dissection

Activity Instructions

1. Put on gloves and get a dissection tray, scalpel, and measuring tape

2. Obtain the mammalian digestive tract and place it on the tray

3. Identify the following structures (note that your preparation may not have the esophagus and/or the accessory organs):
   - Esophagus
   - Stomach
   - Small intestine
   - Large intestine
     - Cecum
   - Rectum
   - Liver
   - Gallbladder
   - Pancreas

Activity Questions

1. Use the measuring tape to measure the length of the stomach, small intestine, large intestine, and rectum of the specimen. Record these lengths in Table 23.4.

2. How do the lengths of the mammal's organs compare with the lengths of human organs?

Table 23.4 Length of Human Organs vs. Other Mammal Organs		
Organ	Length in Human	Length in Other Mammal
Stomach	0.30 m	
Small intestine	3–4 m	
Large intestine	1–1.5 m	
Rectum	0.19 m	

Post-Lab Assessment

1. Which region of the pharynx does not encounter food? Why?

_____

_____

2. List the parts of the GI tract in the order in which they encounter food. Include the regions of organs where applicable (e.g., duodenum of the small intestine).

_____

_____

_____

3. Describe the flow of bile from the gallbladder to the duodenum.

_____

_____

4. Which liver lobe is more superior: the caudate or the quadrate?

_____

5. Describe the structures of the hepatic portal system.

_____

_____

6. What is the function of the villi and microvilli in the epithelium of the small intestine? How do the two differ structurally?

_____

_____

7. **Critical Thinking:** Based on the functions of the stomach and small intestine, what do you think is the difference in function between the rugae and the circular folds?

_____

_____

24

Endocrine System Anatomy and Physiology

Textbook Correlation: Chapter 15—Metabolism and Endocrine Control

Details

Activities	Activity Objectives	Required Materials	Estimated Time
24-1: Endocrine System Anatomy	Identify the endocrine glands on models	• Torso model • Brain model	10 min
24-2: Microscopic Endocrine Anatomy	Identify the microscopic anatomy of endocrine glands and structures	• Microscope • Slides (pancreas, pituitary, adrenal gland, thyroid gland, parathyroid gland)	25 min
24-3: Hormone Quiz Show	Determine the producing gland, target organ(s), and function(s) of hormones	• Quiz game	45 min
24-4: Categorizing Hormones	Apply your knowledge of glands, hormones, targets, and actions in a hormone game		35 min

Overview

The best-known endocrine disorder is diabetes mellitus, which is due to decreased or inhibited functioning of the pancreas. The number of people in the United States diagnosed with type 2 diabetes is skyrocketing at an alarming rate because of poor diet and increasing obesity. It is even diagnosed in young children. The medical community is very concerned about the diabetes epidemic because the complications of diabetes are so serious, and both the disease and its complications are costly to treat. Type 2 diabetes is preventable in many but not all individuals by following a nourishing, balanced diet, exercising, and maintaining the suggested weight for your height and bone structure.

Need to Know

- Endocrine glands: Organs that specialize in the production of chemical messengers called **hormones,** which travel through the bloodstream to alter the activity of **target organs**

- **Pancreas:** located posterior to the stomach and superior to the transverse colon in the upper left quadrant
  - Secretes **insulin** and **glucagon**

- **Pituitary gland:** housed in the sella turcica of the sphenoid bone; extends from the hypothalamus
  - Separated into the
    - Anterior pituitary: synthesizes and secretes **hypophysiotropic hormones**
      - Gonadotropins
      - Prolactin
      - Adrenocorticotropic hormone
      - Thyroid-stimulating hormone
      - Growth hormone
    - Posterior pituitary: extension of the hypothalamus, contains neurons, and secretes
      - Antidiuretic hormone
      - Oxytocin

- **Adrenal gland:** located superior and slightly medial to the kidneys
  - Divided into two regions:
    - Outer **cortex,** which secretes
      - Glucocorticoids
      - Androgen
      - Mineralocorticoids
    - Deep **medulla,** which secretes
      - Epinephrine and norepinephrine

- **Thyroid gland:** butterfly-shaped gland located on the inferior portion of the larynx and the superior portion of the trachea
  - Secretes **thyroxine** and **triiodothyronine**

- **Parathyroid gland:** small glands embedded on the posterior surface of the thyroid gland
  - Secretes **parathyroid hormone**

Pre-Lab Activity

Students should complete this activity before completing the lab activities that follow.

Match the following secreting glands to the correct hormone. Some answers may be used more than once.

A. Adrenal cortex
B. Adrenal medulla
C. Anterior pituitary
D. Pancreas
E. Parathyroid gland
F. Posterior pituitary
G. Thyroid gland

1. This gland secretes prolactin: _____

2. This gland secretes glucocorticoids: _____

3. This gland secretes oxytocin:_____

4. This gland secretes insulin: _____

5. This gland secretes norepinephrine: _____

6. This gland secretes androgens: _____

7. This gland secretes growth hormone:_____

8. This gland secretes parathyroid hormone: _____

9. This gland secretes triiodothyronine: _____

10. This gland secretes adrenocorticotropic hormone: _____

Endocrine System Anatomy

Activity Instructions

On the endocrine models, identify the structures listed in the left-hand column of Table 24.1. As you identify each structure, write down the corresponding number in the right-hand column. Indicate the model in which you located each gland. Use Figures 15.13 and 15.17 in your textbook for reference.

Table 24.1 Endocrine Organs		
Structure	**Model**	**Corresponding Number on the Model**
Adrenal gland		
Hypothalamus		
Pituitary stalk		
Pancreas		
Pituitary gland		
Thyroid gland		

Activity Questions

1. Name the structure that connects the hypothalamus to the pituitary gland.

   _____

   _____

2. Name the glands located on the posterior side of the thyroid gland (not visible on the models).

   _____

   _____

3. Name the gland that is superior to the kidneys.

   _____

   _____

4. Describe the location of the pancreas.

   _____

   _____

   _____

   _____

   _____

   _____

Microscopic Endocrine Anatomy

Activity Instructions

1. Identify the following structures on the pancreas slide under high power. Draw, label, and describe your findings. See Figure 15.14 of the textbook.

   - Pancreatic islets (islets of Langerhans)
     - α-cells (alpha)
     - β-cells (beta)

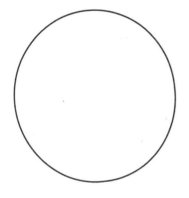

TM _____

Slide name _____

Description _____

_____

_____

_____

_____

2. Identify the following structures on the pituitary gland slide under low power. Draw, label, and describe your findings. See Figure 15.20 of the textbook.
   - Pituitary stalk
   - Anterior pituitary
   - Posterior pituitary

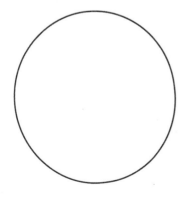

TM _____

Slide name _____

Description _____

_____

_____

_____

TM _____

Slide name _____

Description _____

_____

_____

_____

_____

3. Identify the following structures on the adrenal gland slide under both low and high powers. Draw, label, and describe your findings.
- Cortex
- Medulla

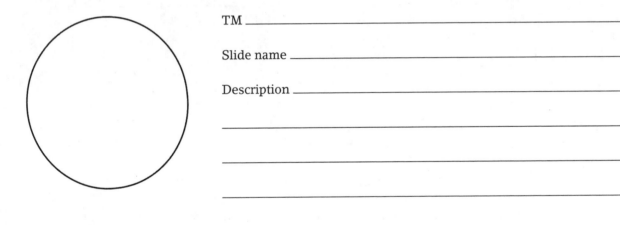

TM _____

Slide name _____

Description _____

_____

_____

_____

4. Identify the following structures on the thyroid gland slide under low power. Draw, label, and describe your findings. See Figure 15.23 of your textbook.
   ● Follicles filled with colloid

TM _____

Slide name _____

Description _____

_____

_____

_____

_____

5. Identify the parathyroid gland slide under high power. Draw, label, and describe your findings.

TM _____

Slide name _____

Description _____

_____

_____

_____

_____

Activity Questions

1. Does the pancreas contain a larger amount of exocrine or endocrine cells?

   _____

   _____

2. Describe the structural differences between the anterior and posterior pituitary gland.

   _____

   _____

   _____

   _____

3. Describe the structural differences between the adrenal cortex and the adrenal medulla.

   _____

   _____

   _____

   _____

4. Describe the structural difference between the thyroid gland and the parathyroid gland.

   _____

   _____

   _____

5. **Critical Thinking:** People with type 1 diabetes are incapable of producing insulin. What cells are not functioning? Be specific.

   _____

   _____

Hormone Quiz Game

This activity allows you to test your knowledge of hormones by playing a Jeopardy-like quiz game.

Activity Instructions

Your instructor will provide specific rules and instructions.

After the game, make notes on the lines below about which concepts you need to study further to master:

_____

_____

_____

_____

_____

_____

_____

_____

_____

_____

_____

_____

_____

_____

_____

_____

_____

_____

Categorizing Hormones

Activity Instructions

In this activity, you will be working in groups in order to categorize glands, hormones, hormone targets, and hormone functions.

Part I: Secreting Glands

1. The names of endocrine glands are written around the room.

2. The instructor will distribute index cards with the names of secreting cells (or regions) written in orange and the names of hormones written in purple.

3. Work together to match the correct secreting cell with the correct glan. Once you think that you have correctly matched the cell with the gland, tape the index card to the wall below the name of the gland.

4. Next, do the same with hormones. Determine the name of the cell (or gland) that secretes each hormone and tape the name of the hormone under the correct cell or gland.
   - As you are working on this activity, the instructor will walk around the room and check your answers. Correct answers will be marked with a check mark. Any incorrect answer will be left unmarked so that you know to move the index card to a different location.

5. Once all index cards have been correctly categorized, answer Activity Question 1.

6. Remove the index cards with the names of the glands and the secreting cells (or regions) and tape the name of the hormone higher up on the wall (or board).

Part II: Hormone Targets and Action

7. The instructor will distribute index cards with the name of target organs written in green and a description of the hormone action in red.

8. Work together to match the target organ(s) or cells to the correct hormone. Tape the index card to the wall under the name of the hormone.

9. Next, do the same with hormone action and tape the card below the target organ.
   - As you are working on this activity, the instructor will walk around the room and check your answers. Correct answers will be marked with a check mark. Any incorrect answer will be left unmarked so that you know to move the index card to a different location.

10. Once all of the index cards have been correctly categorized, answer Activity Question 2.

11. Remove all of the index cards and return them to your instructor.

Activity Questions

1. Complete Table 24.2 using the index cards as a reference. Two of the rows have been filled out for you.

Table 24.2   Glands, Cells, and Hormones

Gland	Secreting Cell or Region	Hormone(s)
Pancreas	α-cells	Glucagon
	β-cells	Insulin
Posterior Pituitary		Anti-diuretic hormone and oxytocin
Anterior Pituitary		
Adrenal gland		
Thyroid gland		
Parathyroid gland		

2. Fill in Table 24.3 using the index cards as a reference. The first row has been filled out for you.

Table 24.3   Hormone Targets and Actions

Hormone	Target(s)	Action(s)
Insulin	Liver, skeletal muscle, adipose tissue	Promotes glucose uptake in adipose and nonexercising skeletal muscle cells, stimulates glycolysis and glycogenesis, inhibits gluconeogenesis and glycogenolysis, stimulates lipogenesis and protein synthesis
Glucagon		
Antidiuretic hormone		
Oxytocin		
Gonadotropins		
Prolactin		
Adrenocorticotropic hormone		
Thyroid-stimulating hormone		
Growth hormone		
Glucocorticoids		
Androgens	Many	
Mineralocorticoids		
Epinephrine and norepinephrine	Many	
Thyroxine and triiodothyronine	Many	
Parathyroid hormone		

Post-Lab Assessment

1. Name the gland and cells that secrete glucagon.

   _____

2. Name one target for parathyroid hormone.

   _____

3. Describe the action of mineralocorticoids.

   _____

   _____

4. Name two hormones secreted by the anterior pituitary.

   _____

5. Name two hormones that target the female mammary gland.

   _____

6. **Critical Thinking:** The gonadotropins stimulate the gonads (testes and ovaries) to produce and secrete hormones. What hormone is produced and secreted by the testes? Which two hormones are produced and secreted by the ovaries?

   _____

   _____

25

Urinary System Anatomy and Urinalysis

Textbook Correlation: Chapter 16—The Urinary System and Body Fluids

Details

Activities	Activity Objectives	Required Materials	Estimated Time
25-1: Urinary System Anatomy	Identify the organs and structures of the urinary system	● Torso (or urinary system model) ● Male pelvic model ● Female pelvic model	20 min
25-2: Kidney Anatomy	Identify the structures and blood vessels of the kidney	● Kidney model ● Nephron model	35 min
25-3: Mammalian Kidney Dissection	Identify the structures and blood vessels on a mammalian (sheep or pig) kidney	● Dissecting pan ● Gloves ● Knife ● Mammalian kidney (pig, sheep, or bovine)	15 min
25-4: Build a Nephron	Identify the structures of a nephron	● Modeling clay (blue, gray, green, orange, purple, red, yellow)	15 min
25-5: Urinalysis	Identify the abnormal contents of urine; determine a possible cause for an abnormal urine sample	● Simulated urine ● Wax pencil ● Test tube rack ● 5 test tubes ● Urine test strips with bottle ● Urinometer ● Magnifying glass	40 min

Overview

Believe it or not, a person can live without a stomach, colon, appendix, gallbladder, or spleen. A person can also thrive with only one functioning kidney. In fact, if one kidney is removed, the remaining kidney will actually increase in size in order to accommodate its additional workload. But what happens if the one remaining kidney becomes diseased or fails to function properly? If toxins cannot be removed from the bloodstream and disposed of in urine, they can build up. The only cure for this is a kidney transplant, and many patients wait years for their names to rise to the top of the transplant waiting list. Patients waiting for their new kidneys must undergo a treatment procedure called dialysis, in which a machine acts like the kidney and filters out the toxins from the blood. One cause of kidney failure that has only recently been recognized is smoking—yet another reason to avoid such a deadly habit.

Today's lab will look at the structure and function of these essential blood-filtering organs as well as other components of the urinary system.

Need to Know

- **Kidneys:** paired organs adhering to the dorsal body wall, lateral to the lower thoracic vertebrae and superior lumbar vertebrae
  - **Renal capsule:** layer of connective tissue that surrounds the kidney
  - **Renal pelvis:** triangular area where urine collects in the kidney
  - **Renal cortex:** outer pale region
  - **Renal medulla:** innermost dark-staining region
    - **Renal pyramids:** triangular (cone-shaped) structures that comprise the renal medulla
    - **Renal papillae:** pointed tips of the pyramids
  - **Calyces:** cup-shaped structures that empty the renal papillae and merge into the renal pelvis

- **Nephron:** structural and functional unit of the kidney; composed of the
  - **Glomerulus:** capillary bed that filters blood to produce **filtrate**
    - The glomerulus is pushed into the proximal tip of the *renal tubule* (see below), like a fingertip pushed into a long balloon.
  - **Renal tubule:** a tube that receives and modifies the filtrate in order to produce urine.
    - **Glomerular capsule:** modified tubule cells forming a compartment surrounding the glomerulus; receives fluid (filtrate) that filters out of blood.
    - **Proximal tubule:** site of maximal reabsorption
    - **Nephron loop:** U-shaped structure that either extends a short way (**cortical nephron**) or a long way (**juxtaglomerular nephron**) into the renal medulla
      - Consists of a descending loop and an ascending loop
      - Establishes an osmotic gradient in the renal medulla that is necessary for producing concentrated urine
    - **Distal tubule:** site of regulated sodium, potassium, and acid reabsorption and/or secretion
    - **Collecting duct:** Site of regulated water absorption; collects the filtrate (now **urine**) from many distal tubules and drains the urine into the calyces

- **Renal blood flow:** oxygen-rich blood enters from the abdominal aorta and oxygen-poor blood exits into the inferior vena cava.
  - **Renal artery:** branches off the abdominal aorta
  - **Arcuate artery:** forms an arc between the renal cortex and medulla
  - **Interlobular artery:** radiates into the cortex
  - **Afferent arteriole:** branches off the interlobular artery and feeds into the glomerulus
  - **Glomerulus:** capillary bed responsible for producing filtrate
  - **Efferent arteriole:** drains blood from the glomerulus
  - **Peritubular capillaries:** capillary bed that is intertwined with the renal tubules; exchanges solutes with the filtrate by reabsorption and secretion
    - ○ **Vasa recta:** branch of the peritubular capillary bed that extends deeply into the medulla
  - **Interlobular vein:** drains the peritubular capillaries
  - **Arcuate vein:** located between the cortex and the medulla
  - **Renal vein:** vessel through which oxygen-poor blood exits the kidney

- **Ureters:** tubes that transport urine from the kidneys to the urinary bladder

- **Urinary bladder:** storage facility for urine
  - **Rugae:** folds in the mucosa of the organ that allow for expansion during urine storage
  - **Detrusor muscle:** layer of muscle in the urinary bladder wall

- **Urethra:** tube that drains urine from the urinary bladder to the external environment
  - **Internal urethral sphincter:** involuntary smooth muscle immediately inferior to the urethral exit from the urinary bladder
  - **External urethral sphincter:** band of voluntary skeletal muscle located several centimeters inferior to the internal urethral sphincter
  - **Urethral orifice:** opening to the external environment

- **Urine**
  - Consists of water, electrolytes, and nitrogenous wastes from protein metabolism (urea, uric acid, ammonia, and creatinine)
  - Specific gravity: density of urine compared with that of distilled (pure) water (1.000)
    - ○ Measured by a urinometer
    - ○ Varies from 1.003 to 1.016
    - ○ Depends on the amount of solutes: dilute (closer to 1.003) or concentrated (1.016)
  - The following substances should *not* be found in urine (presence indicates disorder/disease)
    - ○ Erythrocytes, leukocytes, hemoglobin, bacteria, protein, nitrites, glucose

Pre-Lab Activity

Students should complete this activity before completing the lab activities that follow.

1. Label the kidney structures in the diagram below with the terms used in the need to know section.

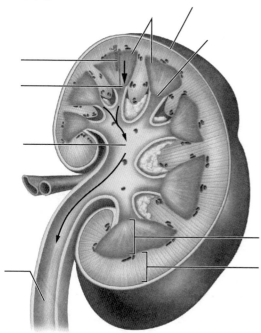

2. Label the parts of urinary bladder in the diagram below using the terms in the need to know section.

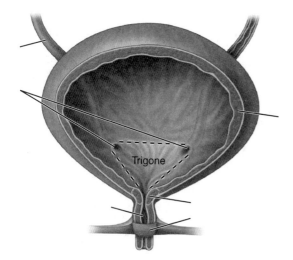

Trigone

3. Color the diagram of the nephron below using the following color code:
   ● Glomerulus: red
   ● Glomerular capsule: brown
   ● Proximal tubule: blue
   ● Nephron loop (descending limb): orange
   ● Nephron loop (ascending limb): green
   ● Distal tubule: yellow
   ● Collecting duct: purple

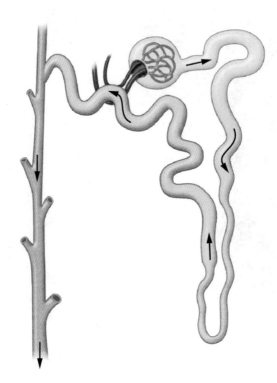

4. List at least four substances that should *not* be found in a urine specimen.

_____

_____

Urinary System Anatomy

Activity Instructions

On the torso and male and female pelvic models, identify the organs and structures listed in the left-hand column of Table 25.1. As you identify each structure, write down the corresponding number in the right-hand column. Write the name of the model in which you identified each structure in the middle column. Refer to Figures 16-3, 16-5, and 17-7 in your textbook.

Table 25.1 Parts of the Urinary System		
Organ/Structure	Model	Corresponding Number on the Model
Kidneys (right and left)		
Ureters (right and left)		
Urinary bladder		
Internal ureteral orifices		
Internal urethral orifice		
Detrusor muscle		
Rugae		
Urethra		
Internal urethral sphincter		
External urethral sphincter		
External urethral orifice		

Activity Questions

1. Name the tubes that connect the kidneys to the urinary bladder.

   _____

2. Which sex has a longer urethra? Why?

   _____

   _____

3. **Critical Thinking:** Rugae were also present in the stomach. Based on the function of the rugae in the stomach, what do you think they do in the urinary bladder?

   _____

   _____

   _____

4. **Critical Thinking:** You may have noticed that the urinary bladder is larger on the male pelvic models than on the female pelvic models. This is anatomically correct. Why do you think that this is true?

   _____

   _____

   _____

5. **Critical Thinking:** Females are more prone to bacterial urinary tract infections, which occur when bacteria enter the urethra and travel to the urinary bladder. Based on the anatomy of the male and female urinary systems, why do you think that females are more vulnerable to urinary tract infections? Hint: Remember that the large intestine contains bacteria.

   _____

   _____

   _____

   _____

Kidney Anatomy

Activity Instructions

On the kidney and nephron models, identify the organs and structures listed in the left-hand column of Tables 25.2, 25.3, and 25.4. As you identify each structure, write down the corresponding number in the right-hand column. Refer to Figures 16.4, 16.6, 16.8, and 16.13 in your textbook.

Table 25.2 Kidney Anatomy	
Structure	**Corresponding Number on the Model**
Capsule	
Renal pelvis	
Cortex	
Medulla	
Renal pyramid	
Renal papillae	
Calyx	
Nephron	

Table 25.3   Nephron Anatomy

Structure	Corresponding Number on the Model
Cortical nephron	
Juxtamedullary nephron	
Glomerular capsule	
Glomerular space	
Glomerulus	
Endothelial cells	
Podocytes with filtration slits	
Proximal tubule	
Nephron loop (loop of Henle)	
Descending limb	
Ascending limb	
Distal tubule	
Collecting duct	
Juxtaglomerular apparatus	
Granular cells	
Macula densa	

Table 25.4 Renal Blood Vessel Anatomy

Blood Vessel	Corresponding Number on the Model
Renal artery	
Arcuate artery	
Interlobular artery	
Afferent arteriole	
Glomerulus	
Efferent arteriole	
Peritubular capillaries	
Vasa recta	
Interlobular vein	
Arcuate vein	
Renal vein	

Activity Questions

1. Name the part of the renal tubule that receives filtrate from the glomerular capsule.

_____

2. Name the structure that delivers urine to the ureter.

_____

3. Describe the difference between a cortical nephron and a juxtamedullary nephron.

_____

_____

4. What is the difference between the *renal medulla* and the *renal pyramids*?

_____

_____

5. Three capillary beds are found in the kidney. Name them.

_____

_____

6. Name the artery that is found at the border of the cortex and medulla.

_____

7. Differentiate between the location of the granular cells and the cells of the macula densa.

_____

_____

Activity 25-3

Mammalian Kidney Dissection

This dissection will allow you to appreciate the structures and blood vessels of a more true-to-life kidney than the models represent. A pig kidney may be used in place of a sheep kidney.

Activity Instructions

1. Obtain a dissecting pan, knife, and gloves.

2. Put the gloves on, get a kidney, and place the kidney in the dissecting pan.

3. Observe the following external structures:
- Adipose tissue
- Capsule

4. Use the knife to make a frontal incision in the kidney.

5. Identify the following internal structures:
   - Renal capsule
   - Renal cortex
   - Renal medulla
     - Medullary pyramid
   - Calyx
   - Renal pelvis
   - Ureter

6. If your kidney is injected, identify the following blood vessels:
   - Renal artery
   - Arcuate artery
   - Interlobular artery
   - Interlobular vein
   - Arcuate vein
   - Renal vein

Note: veins are typically easier to identify than arteries in the injected specimen.

Activity Questions

1. Name the layers of the kidney from superficial to deep.

_____

_____

2. Which structure is located closer to the medullary pyramids: a calyx or the renal pelvis?

_____

_____

3. Name the blood vessels that radiate into the renal cortex.

_____

_____

Build a Nephron

In this activity, you will build a nephron with different colors of modeling clay.

Activity Instructions

1. Get a piece of **red** modeling clay and roll it into a ball.

2. Put small strips of **gray** clay on the red ball, leaving small spaces between the gray clay.

3. Make a cup-shaped structure using **blue** modeling clay and place the red ball with the gray strips in the blue cup that you made.

4. Using a piece of **orange** clay, roll it out into a long cylinder. Attach it to the blue cup and mold curves (like a snake) in the orange cylinder.

5. Obtain a piece of **green** clay. Roll it out into a long cylinder and attach it to the orange tube, and form it into a U.

6. Get a piece of **purple** clay. Roll it out and attach it to the green tube. Make it curvy, as you did with the orange cylinder.

7. Roll a piece of **yellow** clay out into a long tube and attach it to the free end of the purple clay.

Activity Questions

Determine the nephron structure that each color clay represents:

1. Blue: _____

2. Gray: _____

3. Green: _____

4. Orange: _____

5. Purple: _____

6. Red: _____

7. Yellow: _____

Urinalysis

You will act as a lab technician in this laboratory exercise by testing samples of simulated urine for abnormal constituents. You will then read the chart notes of each patient and match the urine sample to the patient.

 Note: This is *not* how it is done in a real clinical setting. Each urine sample obtained is properly labeled with the patient's name so that the nurses and physicians are not matching urine samples to patient complaints/history.

Part I: Data Collection

Activity Instructions

1. Use a wax pencil to label five test tubes A, B, C, D, and E.

2. Pour a small amount of simulated urine from each stock container into each test tube. Be sure to pour stock solution A into the test tube labeled A, B stock into the B test tube, and so on.

3. Get a blank piece of unlined white paper, turn the paper sideways, and draw four vertical lines down the paper so that you have five columns. Label the columns A to E.

4. Get a test strip from the container and close the lid after getting the strip.

5. Dip the strip into the test tube labeled A (contains sample A) quickly and the remove it. Put the strip on the white paper in column A.

6. Look at the test strip container in order to interpret your results. There should be a time frame listed for each variable, which indicates how long you should wait before you interpret your results. Be sure to record your results in Table 25.5 within the time frame; failure to do so can result in a false positive.

7. Repeat steps 4 through 6 for each sample, placing the test strip in the appropriate column. **Important:** Be sure to use a different strip for each sample in order to prevent cross-contamination.

Caution: It is important to get each test strip just before you use it and to put the lid back on the container immediately after getting the strip. The strips are very sensitive to light and humidity.

8. Place a urinometer in test tube A and use a magnifying glass to obtain the reading. Record the results in the table below. Remove the urinometer and rinse it off with deionized (distilled) water. **Important:** It is very important to use distilled water (not tap water) to rinse off the urinometer.

9. Repeat step 8 to test the specific gravity of each sample. Be sure to rinse off the urinometer between samples.

Table 25.5   Urinalysis Data

	Sample A	Sample B	Sample C	Sample D	Sample E
Color of specimen					
Blood (Hb)					
pH					
Leukocytes					
Ketones					
Glucose					
Protein					
Nitrites					
Specific gravity					

Part II: Chart Notes

Activity Instructions

Read the following chart notes of patients who were admitted to the local emergency room. While you are reading the case studies, think about which urine sample best matches each patient scenario.

Patient Rashad Patel in Room 207

Chart Notes: Patient is a 17-year-old slender male who arrived by ambulance from his 14-year-old sister's birthday party at a local park. His parents stated that the patient had eaten two pieces of cake at the party. Parents also stated that the patient had been using the restroom frequently during the party. The parents called for medics when Rashad complained of blurred vision, seemed confused as to where he was, and had very sweet-smelling breath. The patient is a type-1 diabetic. The patient's blood glucose monitor had not been used since several hours earlier.

Patient Kara Billings in Room 215

Chart Notes: Patient is a 21-year-old female who arrived at the emergency room via ambulance after passing out at a local amusement park. Outside temperature was approximately 101°F (39°C). BAC (blood alcohol content) came back at approximately 0.057%, indicating that the patient was consuming alcohol and is moderately intoxicated. Patient is not producing much urine. Urine produced is very dark.

Patient April Lee in Room 235

Chart Notes: Patient is a 46-year-old woman complaining of the frequent, sudden urge to urinate without producing much urine. Rates pain associated with urination at a 5 on a scale of 1 to 10.

Patient Emmanuel Bonvier in Room 222

Chart Notes: Patient is a 6-year-old male; newly arrived immigrant from Haiti. Mother and child do not speak English. Questions and answers were translated by a family friend. Patient's urine is dark brown and cloudy. Patient suffered from a sore throat, high fever, and body aches 2 weeks prior to his symptoms [suspected strep throat]. Emmanuel admitted to hospital for 24 hours observation. Oliguria (low urine output) noted.

    Diagnosis: Glomerulonephritis stemming from strep throat infection.

- Note: This patient might be the hardest to match with urinalysis results. Remember, the suffix *-itis* indicates inflammation, which in this case means that the glomerulus is inflamed. Inflammation of the glomerulus increases capillary permeability.
- Hint: Think about the normal function of the glomerulus.

Activity Questions

1. Which sample was normal? How do you know?

_____

_____

2. Match the patient with the urine sample. One sample will not be used since it is the normal (control) sample.

    a. Sample A   ● Rashad Patel: _____

    b. Sample B

    c. Sample C   ● Kara Billings: _____

    d. Sample D

    e. Sample E   ● April Lee: _____

                ● Emmanual Bonvier: _____

3. Critical Thinking: If not given in the case, determine a diagnosis for each patient based on chart notes and urinalysis. For all cases, explain why the abnormal constituents were found in each urine sample based on the diagnosis.

    a. Rashad Patel (diagnosis known):

_____

_____

_____

_____

b. Kara Billings:

_____

_____

_____

_____

c. April Lee:

_____

_____

_____

_____

d. Emmanuel Bonvier (diagnosis known):

_____

_____

_____

_____

1. Trace the flow of filtrate through the nephron by listing all of the structures that the filtrate will encounter.

   _____

   _____

2. Trace the flow of urine from the collecting duct to the external urethral orifice by listing all of the structures that the urine will encounter.

   _____

   _____

3. Trace blood flow through the kidney from the renal artery to the renal vein by listing all of the structures that the blood will encounter.

   _____

   _____

4. Think about typical capillary beds found throughout the body. They are fed by an arteriole and drained by a venule. How is the glomerulus unique compared with most capillary beds?

   _____

   _____

5. Put an X by the following components that should *not* be found in a normal urine specimen:
   - Water: _____
   - Glucose: _____
   - Protein: _____
   - Sodium ions: _____
   - Urea: _____
   - Erythrocytes: _____
   - Hydrogen ions: _____

6. **Critical Thinking:** Despite the fact that Kara (Activity 25-5) was drinking alcohol, a diuretic, she was not producing much urine. A diuretic is a substance that increases the frequency of urination. Why wasn't she producing much urine? Be sure to include the effect of the increased temperature and hormone action in your answer.

   _____

   _____

   _____

26

Male and Female Reproductive Systems

Textbook Correlation: Chapter 17—The Reproductive System

Details

Activities	Activity Objectives	Required Materials	Estimated Time
26-1: Anatomy of the Male Reproductive System	Identify the organs and structures of the male reproductive system	● Male pelvic model	20 min
26-2: Meiosis Activity	Illustrate the stages of meiosis; identify the number of chromosomes in the gametes during each stage of meiosis	● Modeling clay (yellow, purple, orange)	25 min
26-3: Spermatogenesis and Spermiogenesis	Identify the stages of spermatogenesis and spermiogenesis; determine the number of chromosomes found in each stage; identify the parts of spermatozoa	● Meiosis model ● Microscope ● Testis or spermatogenesis slide ● Sperm slide	20 min
26-4: Anatomy of the Female Reproductive System	Identify the organs and structures of the female reproductive system and breast	● Female pelvic model ● Mammary gland model	30 min
26-5: Ovary and Oogenesis	Identify the parts of an ovary; identify the stages of oogenesis; list the differences between a primary and mature follicle	● Meiosis model ● Ovary model ● Microscope ● Ovary slide	30 min

Overview

Women typically begin going to the gynecologist as teenagers and continue annual appointments throughout their lives. One of the procedures performed during every annual exam is a Pap smear, during which the physician extracts a scraping of cervical cells for observation. The physician is looking for abnormal cervical cells, typically caused by human papillomavirus (HPV), which can develop into cancer. HPV is a very common sexually transmitted disease (STD) and often is not accompanied by any signs or symptoms. Where is the cervix? Do males have a cervix? These are some of the questions that you will answer today in exploring the male and female reproductive systems.

Need to Know

- **Male Reproduction System**
  - **Testes:** male gonads
    - **Leydig cells** produce testosterone
    - **Seminiferous tubules** produce spermatozoa (the male *gametes*, or sex cells)
    - Located outside of the body and enclosed by the **scrotum**
  - **Ducts:** convey sperm from tubules to environment
    - **Epididymis:** highly coiled structure located posteriorly to each testis; stores sperm
    - **Ductus (vas) deferens:** receives sperm from the epididymis during ejaculation
    - **Ejaculatory duct:** transfers semen from the ductus deferens to the urethra
    - **Urethra:** transfers urine or sperm (not simultaneously) externally
  - **Glands** produce the liquid portion of semen.
    - **Seminal vesicles:** honeycomb-shaped glands located on the sides of the urinary bladder
    - **Prostate gland:** plum-shaped structure inferior to the urinary bladder
    - **Bulbourethral glands:** small pea-shaped glands; ducts empty into the urethra
  - **Penis:** male organ of copulation
    - **Corpora cavernosa:** paired dorsal erectile tissue
    - **Corpus spongiosum:** ventral erectile tissue

- **Female Reproductive System**
  - **Clitoris:** erectile tissue located anterior to the vaginal introitus (opening)
  - **Vagina:** female organ of copulation, located posterior to the urethra and anterior to the rectum
  - **Uterus:** large organ superior and posterior to the urinary bladder
    - Protects and provides nutrients for the fetus
    - **Cervix:** entrance to the uterus
    - **Endometrium:** lines the uterine cavity; partially shed during menstruation
    - **Myometrium:** thick muscular layer
  - **Ovaries:** female gonads
    - Produce oocytes (female gametes) and female sex steroids (estrogen and progesterone)
    - **Follicles** protect oocytes and secrete sex steroids
  - **Uterine tubes:** carry oocytes from the ovary to the uterus
  - **Mammary glands:** exocrine glands located in the breasts that produce and secrete milk in lactating females

- **Meiosis**
  - Specialized process of cell division that occurs only to produce gametes
  - Consists of two cell divisions:
    - ○ Begins with one **diploid** (46 chromosomes) stem cell
    - ○ Ends with four **haploid** (23 chromosomes) genetically unique daughter cells
  - **Spermatogenesis:** production of spermatozoa; occurs in the seminiferous tubules of the testes
    - ○ **Spermatogonia** (stem cells) are located adjacent to the tubule wall.
    - ○ **Mitosis:** each spermatogonium divides into two identical cells; one remains as a spermatogonium and the other differentiates into a **primary spermatocyte** (2n, or diploid).
    - ○ **Meiosis I:** each primary spermatocyte divides to produce two haploid **secondary spermatocytes.**
    - ○ **Meiosis II:** each secondary spermatocyte divides, forming a total of four haploid **spermatids.**
    - ○ **Spermiogenesis:** spermatids differentiate into mature spermatozoa.
  - **Oogenesis:** oocyte production; occurs in the ovaries
    - ○ **Oogonia** (stem cells) present only in fetal ovary
    - ○ **Mitosis:** oogonia divide to produce more diploid oogonia
      - ■ Before birth, *all* oogonia differentiate into diploid **primary oocytes**
    - ○ **Meiosis I:** beginning at puberty, each month one primary oocyte completes meiosis I, forming the haploid **secondary oocyte** and a nonfunctional polar body.
      - ■ The secondary oocyte is released from the ovary (**ovulation**).
    - ○ **Meiosis II:** only fertilized secondary oocytes complete meiosis II, forming one zygote (after fusion with sperm nucleus) and one polar body.
  - **Folliculogenesis:** changes in the cells surrounding the oocyte
    - ○ **Primary follicle:** surrounds primary oocytes
    - ○ **Mature follicle:** surrounds secondary oocytes ready for ovulation; contains a cavity (antrum)
    - ○ **Corpus luteum:** follicle converts to this gland after ovulation

Pre-Lab Activity

Students should complete this activity before completing the lab activities that follow.

1. Color the organs in the diagram below according to the following color key:
   - Bulbourethral gland: magenta
   - Ductus deferens: orange
   - Ejaculatory duct: green
   - Epididymis: blue
   - Membranous urethra: black
   - Penile urethra: light green
   - Penis: light blue
   - Prostate: gray
   - Prostatic urethra: pink
   - Rectum: brown
   - Seminal vesicle: purple
   - Testes: red
   - Urinary bladder: yellow

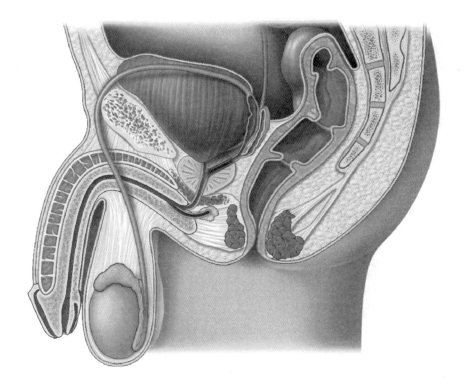

2. Which of the organs in the diagram above is *not* part of the male reproductive system?

_____

3. Color the diagrams below according to the following color key:
- Cervix: yellow
- Clitoris: red
- Ovary: pink
- Rectum: brown
- Urinary bladder: yellow
- Uterine tube: orange
- Uterus: purple
- Vagina: green

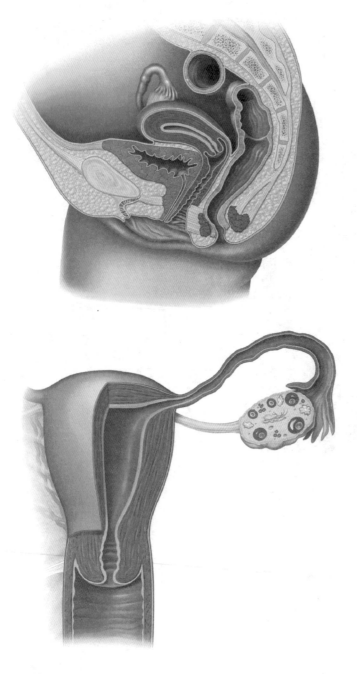

Anatomy of the Male Reproductive System

Activity Instructions

On the male pelvic model, identify the organs and structures listed in the left-hand column of Table 26.1. As you identify each structure, write down the corresponding number in the right-hand column. Refer to Figures 17-1, 17-2, and 17-3 in your textbook.

Table 26.1 Male Reproductive Structures	
Organ/Structure	Corresponding Number on the Model
Scrotum	
Testes	
Epididymis	
Spermatic cord	
Ductus (vas) deferens	
Ejaculatory duct	
Seminal vesicle	
Prostate gland	
Bulbourethral gland	
Prostatic urethra	
Membranous urethra	
Spongy (penile) urethra	

(continued)

Table 26.1 Male Reproductive Structures (continued)	
Organ/Structure	Corresponding Number on the Model
Root (penis)	
Shaft (penis)	
Corpus cavernosum	
Corpus spongiosum	
Glans	
External urethral orifice	

Activity Questions

1. Name the sac of skin that is superficial to the testes.

2. Name the dorsal erectile tissue in the penis.

3. Name the region of the urethra that is the longest.

4. Name the highly coiled structure that is located close to the testes.

5. Name two fluids that exit from the external urethral orifice.

6. Name the structure that connects the ductus deferens to the prostate gland.

7. Name the male gonad.

_____

8. Name the male copulatory organ.

_____

Meiosis Activity

In this activity, you will use modeling clay to represent the movement of chromosomes that occurs in meiosis. Refer to Figures 17-4 and 17-10 in your textbook.

Activity Instructions

1. Get large amount of **yellow** modeling clay and flatten in out like a pancake. This represents a gamete.

2. Get some **purple** and **orange** modeling clay and pinch off a small amount. Roll two strands of each color and place them in the center of the cell. Match up the two same-color strands to form an X (these are called **replicated chromosomes**). Answer Activity Question 1.

3. Line up the replicated chromosomes in the middle of the cell. Remove a small piece of clay from one tip of the purple replicated chromosome. Do the same for the adjacent orange replicated chromosome. Place the small piece of orange clay on the tip of the purple replicated chromosome and put the small piece of purple clay on the tip of the orange replicated chromosome. This represents **crossing over.**

4. Split the large cell into two separate cells, one cell with the purple replicated chromosome and the other cell with the orange replicated chromosome. The cell has now completed **meiosis I.** Answer Activity Questions 2 through 4.

5. Move the replicated chromosomes to the center of each cell.

6. Split each replicated chromosome into individual chromosomes and place them at **opposite** ends of the cell.

7. Split each cell in half. Answer the rest of the activity questions.

Activity Questions

1. If you were making a real human cell, how many replicated chromosomes would you place in the nucleus just before meiosis begins?

   _____

2. How many cells have been produced at the end of meiosis I?

   _____

3. How many replicated chromosomes does each new cell have at the end of meiosis I?

   _____

4. The end result of meiosis is four new gametes. What needs to happen after meiosis I is complete in order to produce two more cells?

   _____

5. Are the newly produced cells diploid or haploid? Explain your answer.

   _____

6. Name two cells that undergo meiosis.

   _____

Activity 26-3

Spermatogenesis and Spermiogenesis

Activity Instructions

1. On the meiosis model, identify the stages of spermatogenesis and spermiogenesis listed in the left-hand column of Table 26.2. As you identify each structure, write down the corresponding number in the right-hand column. Indicate whether the cell is diploid or haploid in the middle column. Refer to Figures 17.3 and 17.4 in your textbook.

Table 26.2   Male Gametes

Stage	Diploid or Haploid	Corresponding Number on the Model
Spermatogonium		
Primary spermatocyte		
Secondary spermatocyte		
Spermatid		
Spermatozoan		
Head	Not applicable	
Midpiece	Not applicable	
Tail (flagellum)	Not applicable	

2. Obtain a microscope slide of a testis (or spermatogenesis) and identify the following structures using low and high power as well as oil immersion. Draw, label, and describe your findings. Refer to Figure 17-3 in your textbook.
   - Seminiferous tubules
   - Developing spermatocytes
   - Spermatozoa
   - Sertoli (sustentacular) cells
   - Leydig (interstitial) cells

TM _____

Slide name _____

Description _____

_____

_____

_____

_____

TM _____

Slide name _____

Description _____

_____

_____

_____

_____

TM _____

Slide name _____

Description _____

_____

_____

_____

_____

3. Obtain a slide of sperm and identify the following structures under high power. Draw, label, and describe your findings. Refer to Figure 17-4 in your textbook.
   - Head
   - Midpiece
   - Tail

TM _____

Slide name _____

Description _____

_____

_____

_____

_____

Activity Questions

1. How many primary spermatocytes result when the spermatogonium divides? How many secondary spermatocytes result when the primary spermatocyte divides? How many spermatids are there after the secondary spermatocytes divide?

_____

_____

2. What is the last cell that is diploid during spermatogenesis?

_____

3. Where in the testis does spermatogenesis occur?

_____

4. Differentiate between the location of the Sertoli cells and that of the Leydig cells.

_____

5. Name the longest part (extension) of the sperm. What is the function of this long process?

_____

Activity 26-4

Anatomy of the Female Reproductive System

Activity Instructions

1. On the female pelvic model, identify the organs and structures listed in the left-hand column of Table 26-3. As you identify each structure, write down the corresponding number in the right-hand column. Refer to Figures 17-6 and 17-7 in your textbook.

Table 26.3 Female Reproductive Structures

Organ/Structure	Corresponding Number on Model
Mons pubis	
Clitoris	
Labia majora	
Labia minora	
Vaginal introitus	
Vestibular glands	
Vagina	
Vaginal fornix	
Cervical os	
Cervical canal	
Uterus body	
Myometrium	
Endometrium	
Endometrial cavity	

Table 26.3   Female Reproductive Structures (continued)

Organ/Structure	Corresponding Number on Model
Uterine tubes	
Ampulla	
Isthmus	
Infundibulum	
Fimbriae	
Ovaries	

2. On the mammary gland model, identify the structures listed in the left-hand column of Table 26.4. As you identify each structure, write down the corresponding number in the right-hand column. Refer to Figure 17-13 in your textbook.

Table 26.4   Mammary Gland Structures

Structure	Corresponding Number on the Model
Lobe	
Lobule	
Lactiferous duct	
Lactiferous sinus	
Nipple	
Areola	
Fat	

Activity Questions

1. Name the erectile organ in the female.

   _____

2. Name the structures that convey gametes between the ovaries and the uterus.

   _____

3. Describe the location of the cervix.

   _____

4. Which uterine wall layer is more superficial: the myometrium or the endometrium?

   _____

5. Name the fingerlike projections of the infundibulum.

   _____

6. Name the female gonad.

   _____

7. Name the female copulatory organ.

   _____

8. Which structure does milk pass through first in a lactating female: the lactiferous duct or the lactiferous sinus?

   _____

9. Name the darkly pigmented area of the breast.

   _____

Ovary and Oogenesis

Activity Instructions

1. On the ovary model, identify the parts of the ovary listed in the left-hand column of Table 26.5. As you identify each structure, write down the corresponding number in the right-hand column. Refer to Figure 17-8 in your textbook.

Table 26.5 Structures of the Ovary	
Structure	**Corresponding Number on the Model**
Germinal epithelium	
Cortex	
Medulla	

2. On the meiosis and ovary model, identify the structures and stages of follicular development and oogenesis listed in the left-hand column of Table 26.6. As you identify each structure, write down the corresponding number in the right-hand column. Refer to Figures 17-8 and 17-10 in your textbook.

Table 26.6 Follicular and Oocyte Development	
Stage	**Corresponding Number on the Model**
Primary follicle	
Follicular cells	
Primary oocyte	
Developing follicle	
Antrum	

(continued)

Table 26-6   Follicular and Oocyte Development (continued)

Stage	Corresponding Number on the Model
Polar body	
Mature follicle	
Secondary oocyte	
Antrum	
Ovulation	
Secondary oocyte	
Corona radiata	
Corpus luteum	
Corpus albicans	

3. Identify the following structures on the ovary slide under both low and high powers. Draw, label, and describe your findings. Refer to Figures 17-8 and 17-10 in your textbook.
   - Primary follicle with primary oocyte
   - Developing follicle with antrum
   - Mature follicle with secondary oocyte and antrum

TM _____

Slide name _____

Description _____

_____

_____

_____

_____

TM _____

Slide name _____

Description _____

_____

_____

_____

TM _____

Slide name _____

Description _____

_____

_____

_____

Activity Questions

1. Where in the ovary does follicular development occur?

_____

2. Which oocyte is haploid: a primary oocyte or a secondary oocyte?

_____

3. When the primary oocyte undergoes division, it produces an oocyte and a nonfunctional cell. What is the name of the nonfunctional cell?

_____

4. What happens to the corpus luteum if fertilization does not occur?

_____

_____

5. Describe how a primary follicle differs from a mature follicle when it is viewed microscopically.

_____

_____

_____

Post-Lab Assessment

1. Trace the flow of sperm from the testes to the external urethral orifice.

   _____

   _____

   _____

2. Why is the urethra considered part of the male reproductive system but not part of the female reproductive system?

   _____

   _____

3. Which cell do you think is smaller: an ovum or a spermatozoan? Why? Relate your answer to the function of each cell.

   _____

   _____

   _____

4. How many functional spermatozoa are there when meiosis is complete? How many functional ova are there after meiosis is complete?

   _____

5. Do all primary spermatocytes complete all phases of meiosis? Do all primary oocytes complete all phases of meiosis? Explain your answer.

   _____

   _____

   _____

   _____

6. **Critical Thinking:** The uterus incubates the growing fetus. One of the many uncomfortable symptoms in the last trimester of pregnancy is a constant urge to urinate. Describe, anatomically, why that occurs.

_____

_____

_____

_____

7. **Critical Thinking:** Why do you think crossing over occurs during meiosis? Why is it important that it should occur?

_____

_____

_____

_____

27

Embryology and Inheritance

Textbook Correlation: Chapter 17—The Reproductive System;
Chapter 18—Life

Details

Activities	Activity Objectives	Required Materials	Estimated Time
27-1: Embryology	Identify the stages of embryonic development and the structures of the growing embryo	● Embryology model set	15 min
27-2: Build a Developing Embryo	Simulate embryonic development using modeling clay	● Modeling clay (yellow, green, blue, red, purple, orange, pink)	25 min
27-3: Heredity	Demonstrate concepts involved in inheritance using a Punnett square	None	40 min
27-4: Pedigrees	Construct and interpret a pedigree	None	20 min

Overview

Shauna had just seen a photograph of her friend Emily's sister. "Wow! You and your sister look almost identical, but my sister and I don't even look like we're related. We have completely different color eyes and hair, she has beautiful curly hair and mine is straight, and she's tall and I'm short!" Emily had just finished a course in anatomy and physiology, so she explained to Shauna about genetics and inheritance patterns. Using Punnett squares, she showed Shauna how a trait like curly hair is passed on. Afterwards, Shauna began thinking about how much she resembled her mom's side of the family and her sister resembled her dad's side of the family. In today's lab you will get to explore the fascinating world of genetics (the study of how traits are passed on) after you look at where it all begins: in the embryo.

Need to Know

- **Gestation:** the duration of pregnancy, conveniently dated from the last menstrual period, which is divided into the:
  - **Embryonic stage:** period of development from *fertilization* (when the sperm nucleus fuses with the ovum nucleus) through the eighth week of gestation
  - **Fetal stage:** period of development from the ninth week of gestation until birth

- Stages in early development:
  - **Zygote:** occurs immediately after fertilization
    - ○ Zygote divides by mitosis into identical daughter cells called **blastomeres**
  - **Blastocyst:** after 4 to 5 days, blastomeres begin to differentiate and migrate, forming the blastocyst, which contains the:
    - ○ **Blastocyst cavity:** hollow cavity
    - ○ **Trophoblast cells:** form the wall of the hollow cavity
    - ○ **Inner cell mass:** group of cells that protrudes into the blastocyst cavity
  - **Implantation:** blastocyst implants in the endometrium of the uterus
  - Differentiation of the inner cell mass:
    - ○ Cells farther from the cavity differentiate into **epiblasts.**
      - ■ **Amniotic cavity** forms within epiblasts
    - ○ Cells closer to the cavity differentiate into **hypoblasts,** which coat the blastocyst wall and the epiblasts.
    - ○ **Yolk sac** takes the place of the blastocyst cavity
  - Formation of the **embryonic plate:**
    - ○ Epiblasts differentiate into three primary germ layers.
      - ■ **Ectoderm:** adjacent to amniotic cavity, forms "outer" tissues such as skin
      - ■ **Mesoderm:** middle layer, forms "middle" tissues such as the muscles
      - ■ **Endoderm:** replaces hypoblasts overlying the inner cell mass, forms "inner" tissues such as the lungs

- **Heredity (genetics):** Passing traits to offspring
  - **Genes:** segments of DNA that code for certain traits (such as eye color, blood type, freckles, etc.)
    - ○ You receive one **allele** (gene version) for each trait from mom and one from dad. This is called your **genotype.**
      - ■ **Phenotype:** the physical expression of the gene (for instance, curly hair or albinism)
    - ○ **Dominant allele:**
      - ■ "Strong" allele; always affects the phenotype regardless of the other allele
      - ■ Indicated by a capital letter

- ○ **Recessive allele:**
    - ▪ Weak allele; affects the phenotype only if there are two recessive alleles
    - ▪ Indicated by a lowercase letter
- ○ **Homozygous:** genotype with two dominant (*DD*) or two recessive (*dd*) alleles
- ○ **Heterozygous:** genotype with one dominant and one recessive (*Dd*) allele; the dominant allele would determine phenotype.
    - ▪ Considered **carriers** in recessive diseases since they can pass the disease to offspring.
- ● **Punnett squares:** can be used to predict the probability of passing a trait or disease to offspring
- ● **Pedigrees:** used to trace traits through the generations
- ● Disorder inheritance patterns:
    - ○ **Autosomal disorders:** disorders that are located on autosomes
        - ▪ **Autosomal recessive:** individual with the disease is homozygous recessive
            - ☐ Carriers are heterozygous.
        - ▪ **Autosomal dominant:** individual with the disease is heterozygous or homozygous dominant.
            - ☐ No carriers
    - ○ **X-linked recessive disorders:** recessive disorders encoded by genes on the X-chromosome
        - ▪ Very common in males, who have only one X chromosome.
        - ▪ Females (two X chromosomes) are commonly carriers.

Pre-Lab Activity

Students should complete this activity before completing the lab activities that follow.

1. Color the diagram below according to the color key:
   - Inner cell mass: red
   - Trophoblasts: green
   - Label the blastocyst cavity.

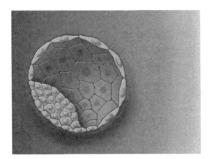

2. Color the diagram below according to the color key:
   - Epiblasts: pink
   - Hypoblasts: yellow
   - Amnion: brown
   - Label the yolk sac and amniotic cavity.

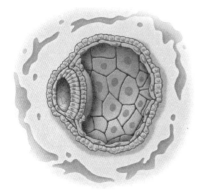

3. Which of the following represents a homozygous recessive genotype: HH, Hh, or hh?

_____

4. What does each of the other genotypes represent?

_____

_____

5. How is a genotype different from a phenotype?

_____

_____

Embryology

Activity Instructions

On the embryology models, identify the embryonic stages and structures listed in the left-hand column of Table 27.1. As you identify each structure, write down the corresponding number in the right-hand column. See Figures 17-14 and 17-15 in the textbook for more information.

Table 27.1	
Stage or Structure	**Corresponding Number on the Model**
Fertilization	
Zygote	
Blastomeres	
Blastocyst (first stage)	
Trophoblast cells	
Inner cell mass	
Blastocyst cavity	
Trophoblast cords (chorion)	
Blastocyst (second stage)	
Hypoblasts	
Epiblasts	
Yolk sac	
Amnion	
Amniotic cavity	

Activity Questions

1. Describe the difference between a zygote and a blastocyst.

_____

_____

2. Which cells develop from the inner cell mass?

_____

3. During which stage of embryonic development does the embryo implant in the uterine wall?

_____

Activity 27-2

Build a Developing Embryo

You will use modeling clay to demonstrate the embryonic stages. Use Figures 17-14 and 17-15 of the textbook to help you identify the structures you are building.

Activity Instructions and Questions

1. Shape some **yellow** modeling clay into a large ball to represent an **ovum**. Use **green** modeling clay to make a small sperm. Insert the head of the sperm into the ovum. Which event just occurred? Where, specifically, did the event occur in the female reproductive tract?

_____

_____

2. Discard the sperm tail and divide the zygote into smaller cells. What are the dividing cells called?

_____

3. Next, illustrate the development of trophoblasts and the inner cell mass. Cut the ball, now called the **blastocyst**, in half and hollow out the center so that you are looking at a section of it. Attach a small amount of **purple** modeling clay to the lining of the hollow cavity. What does the purple modeling clay represent?

_____

4. Next, illustrate the differentiation of hypoblasts and epiblasts and the formation of the amniotic and yolk sac cavities. Replace the purple clay as follows: attach **blue** modeling clay where the purple clay was. Remove the center of the blue clay to make a hollow space. Next, place a layer of **red** clay superior to the blue clay, facing the large hollow space. Stretch the red clay so that it completely lines the large hollow space.
   a. Which color of clay represents the hypoblasts, and which color represents the epiblasts?

   _____

   b. Which cavity (amniotic cavity or yolk sac) is surrounded by the blue clay, and which cavity is surrounded by the red clay?

   _____

5. Finally, illustrate the formation of the three primary germ layers of the embryonic plate. There should be a region between the two cavities where the blue and red clay touch each other, with a small cavity on one side and a large cavity on the other. Replace these *two* layers with *three* new layers; **green**, **pink**, and **orange**. The green layer forms part of the wall of the small cavity, the pink layer is in the middle, and the yellow layer forms part of the wall of the larger cavity. What does each color of the embryonic plate represent?

   a. green: _____

   b. pink: _____

   c. yellow: _____

Inherited Traits and Diseases

Activity Instructions

Work through the example below and then solve the following genetics problems using Punnett squares. Remember that Punnett squares illustrate all of the possible genotypes resulting from a particular mating.

Example: Patrick is heterozygous for albinism (lack of skin pigmentation) and his wife, Marsha, is an albino, which is an autosomal recessive trait. What are the chances that their children will lack skin pigmentation?

Step 1: Determine the genotype for each person and write it down.

Patrick: *Aa*

Marsha: *aa* (must be homozygous recessive since albinism is a recessive trait)

Step 2: Make a table with nine boxes. Put one allele from Patrick in the top center box and the second allele in the top right box. Put Marsha's alleles in the middle and lower boxes on the left (one allele in each box).

	A	**a**
a		
a		

Step 3: Fill in the four empty boxes by combining the alleles.

	A	a
a	**Aa**	**aa**
a	**Aa**	**aa**

Step 4: Answer the question based on the results in the Punnett square.

	A	a
a	Aa	**aa**
a	Aa	**aa**

There is a 50% chance that their offspring will lack pigmentation (albinism), because two out of the four boxes contain the genotype aa.

Activity Questions: Genetics Problems

1. Normal vision is a recessive trait, whereas astigmatism is a dominant one. Annette has normal vision and her husband, Charles, has astigmatism. He has one child from a previous marriage who has normal vision. Use the space below to assemble a Punnett Square.

   a. What is Charles's genotype for astigmatism? Explain your answer.

   _____

   _____

   _____

   b. Annette and Charles are expecting their first baby together. What are the chances that this child will have astigmatism?

   _____

2. Susie has curly hair, which is a dominant trait. Both of her parents have curly hair and all of her siblings have curly hair. Susie married Alan, who has straight hair. Use the space below to assemble a Punnett Square.

a. What is Susie's genotype for curly hair? What is Alan's genotype for straight hair? Is there more than one possible genotype for either person? Explain your answer.

_____

_____

_____

_____

b. What are the possible genotypes and phenotypes for their children?

_____

3. Neither Thomas nor Deidre have cystic fibrosis, yet both of their children have been diagnosed with the disease. Cystic fibrosis is an autosomal recessive disorder. How is it possible that the parents do not have the disease but both children do? Note: The children are genetically related to both parents. Use the space below to assemble a Punnett square, and answer the question on the blank lines.

_____

_____

_____

4. Maria has freckles, which is a dominant trait. What are all of the possible phenotypes of her parents?

_____

_____

_____

5. Huntington's disease is an autosomal dominant disorder. Howard was diagnosed with the disease and is heterozygous. His wife was also genetically tested and she is homozygous recessive. What are the chances that their son will be diagnosed with Huntington's when he becomes older? Use the space below to assemble a Punnett square, and answer the question on the blank lines.

_____

_____

6. Color blindness is an X-linked recessive disorder. Laura is heterozygous for the disorder and her husband Richard is recessive. Use the space below to assemble a Punnett square.

   a. Is Laura's husband color blind?

   _____

   b. What are the chances of Laura and Richard having a color-blind son? A color-blind daughter? If they have a daughter, what are the chances that she will be neither color blind nor a carrier?

   _____

Pedigrees

See Figures 18-2 and 18-3 in the textbook for examples of pedigrees. Remember that geneticists use well-defined symbols in the construction of pedigrees.

1. A female is represented by a circle.

2. A male is represented by a square.

3. A filled-in circle or square indicates that the individual has the trait/disease in question.

4. A half-filled circle or square indicates that the individual is heterozygous (a carrier) for the trait/disease.

5. An empty circle/square indicates that the individual does not have the disease/trait.

6. Horizontal lines between symbols indicate matings; a vertical line descending from this horizontal line indicates offspring. The vertical line branches to indicate multiple offspring.

Activity Instructions

Follow the rules above to construct a pedigree for this case study.

Hemophilia is an autosomal recessive disorder that impairs blood clotting. Aidan has hemophilia. Neither of his parents are hemophiliacs but his maternal grandfather did have hemophilia. Aidan has two siblings. Tony, his brother, is not a hemophiliac and none of Tony's five children is a hemophiliac. Julia, his sister, is not a hemophiliac, but Julia's son is a hemophiliac.

Activity Questions.

1. True or False: Julia's husband *must* be a hemophiliac. Explain your answer.

_____

2. If Aidan marries a woman who is not a hemophiliac and her family has no history of hemophilia, what are the possible genotypes and phenotypes for their offspring?

_____

_____

Post-Lab Assessment

1. Fill in the blanks regarding the stages of embryonic development.

   It begins with _____ (sperm entering the ovum) in the ampulla of the _____

   _____ . The nuclei of the two gametes join, forming a _____, which under-

   goes several mitotic divisions. These divisions results in genetically identical daughter cells,

   which are called the _____. Between days 4 and 5, it is now termed a _____

   and the identical blastomeres begin to differentiate. A blastocyst cavity forms and is lined by

   _____ cells. An _____ _____ _____ forms in a portion of

   the blastocyst cavity, which differentiates into the _____, which hollows out and

   forms the amniotic cavity and the _____, which lines the yolk sac. Eventually, an em-

   bryonic plate forms consisting of three primary germ layers called the _____,

   _____, and _____.

2. **Critical Thinking:** Can there be carriers for autosomal dominant disorders? Explain your
   answer.

   _____

   _____

   _____

3. **Critical Thinking:** Why are males more likely than females to express an X-linked
   recessive trait?

   _____

   _____

   _____

   _____